Leadership and Management of Clinical Trials in Creative Arts Therapy

"Everyone involved in clinical trials should read this brilliant much needed book. Uniquely, Felicity Baker provides an intensive and practical guide, aimed at arts therapists and other allied health professions. Through vivid examples, she leads the reader through the highs and lows of delivering a trial, with solutions, and detailed reflections learned from practice in teams worldwide. This will appeal to all, across the medical, health, creative and social fields."
—Professor Helen Odell-Miller, *OBE Anglia Ruskin University*

"In *Leadership and Management of Clinical Trials in Creative Arts Therapies*, Professor Felicity Baker offers a detailed account of "how to" implement robust large-scale fully-powered clinical trials that meet the rigor required by competitive funding bodies, high impact journals, and policy makers. This timely book is an asset for novice and advanced researchers alike, not only from the creative arts therapies but also from other health professions who want to conduct quality research that can have both clinical impact and policy-changing influences."
—Professor Hod Orkibi, *Ph.D., University of Haifa, Israel*

"This book opens new ground for research in arts therapies and beyond. By discussing the challenges and opportunities of conducting clinical trials in the field of arts therapies, it boosts research in methodologies less used, supporting our intuitive arguments that arts therapies work. For dance movement therapists in particular, it offers a primer of how to navigate around the world of high quality, multi-disciplinary and world-leading research. Its appeal, however, is expected to reach audiences above and beyond researchers in arts therapies. Felicity's in-depth understanding of conducting clinical trials will act as a beacon of good practice for any health professional interested in conducting outcome studies in their discipline."
—Professor Vicky Karkou, *Dance Movement Psychotherapist, Edge Hill University, UK*

"It is well recognized that clinical trials play an important role in the evaluation of care practices and the evolution of health policy. However, the benefits of clinical trials depend on well organized team management, implementation, and knowledge translation. This comprehensive text on leading and managing clinical trials in the creative arts therapies equips researchers with practical skills, clearly documented examples, and an appreciation for interdisciplinary collaboration. It is essential reading for advanced students and researchers in the creative arts therapies."

—Professor Nisha Sajnani, *Chair, Creative Arts Therapies Consortium and International Research Alliance, New York University*

Felicity Anne Baker

Leadership and Management of Clinical Trials in Creative Arts Therapy

Foreword by Christopher Bailey

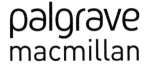

Felicity Anne Baker
The University of Melbourne
Melbourne, VIC, Australia

ISBN 978-3-031-18087-3   ISBN 978-3-031-18085-9 (eBook)
https://doi.org/10.1007/978-3-031-18085-9

© The Editor(s) (if applicable) and The Author(s), under exclusive license to Springer Nature Switzerland AG 2022

This work is subject to copyright. All rights are solely and exclusively licensed by the Publisher, whether the whole or part of the material is concerned, specifically the rights of translation, reprinting, reuse of illustrations, recitation, broadcasting, reproduction on microfilms or in any other physical way, and transmission or information storage and retrieval, electronic adaptation, computer software, or by similar or dissimilar methodology now known or hereafter developed.

The use of general descriptive names, registered names, trademarks, service marks, etc. in this publication does not imply, even in the absence of a specific statement, that such names are exempt from the relevant protective laws and regulations and therefore free for general use.

The publisher, the authors, and the editors are safe to assume that the advice and information in this book are believed to be true and accurate at the date of publication. Neither the publisher nor the authors or the editors give a warranty, expressed or implied, with respect to the material contained herein or for any errors or omissions that may have been made. The publisher remains neutral with regard to jurisdictional claims in published maps and institutional affiliations.

Cover credit: Maram_shutterstock.com

This Palgrave Macmillan imprint is published by the registered company Springer Nature Switzerland AG
The registered company address is: Gewerbestrasse 11, 6330 Cham, Switzerland

Foreword

In the parlance of Knowledge Management, there are two types of knowledge: explicit and tacit. Explicit knowledge is the world of data, information, and evidence. Quantifiable, repeatable, and proven. Tacit knowledge is the world of experience, and if one accumulates enough on a given subject, one can eventually be awarded with the informal distinction of being "wise".

Professor Baker's world is that of explicit knowledge. With over 30 years of practice as one of the world's leading researchers in arts therapies, she has devoted her career to building the evidence base for what works and what does not in this space through rigorous study design and often at scale, as well as publishing the findings in peer reviewed journals with high impact factors, and taking those findings and transforming them into scalable practice, informing national policy in Australia, her base of operations, along the way.

For all her accomplishments in explicit knowledge, this book is not one of them.

This book is an example of tacit knowledge, the accumulated and hard-won wisdom gained from painful experience on how to build the evidence base and bridge that knowledge to scalable implementation. This "how to" book is not about data and evidence, but how to go about building up an evidence base founded on data. How to set up the framework, how to manage the project and budget, and how to disseminate and apply the findings in the real world.

This is an Arts and Health research cookbook. And welcome it is.

From my vantage point at the World Health Organization as the Arts and Health Lead based in Geneva, even a cursory scan of the evidence of the field reveals a plethora of smallish studies, often with grand conclusions associated with them, which from a WHO point of view often don't pass muster as evidence. As intrigued as we are by the possibility of the health benefits of the arts, quantity of small poorly designed studies does not add up to a stronger argument. Anecdote is not the singular of data.

Professor Baker's book may well provide the tools needed for researchers to make a great leap forward in building the evidence base of Arts and Health at a time when our fractious war and disease weary world needs the arts more than ever, but also needs the certainty of scientific method so that we are not unintentionally contributing to the growing cloud of fabulist misinformation which inevitably appears alongside war and disease.

But to understand why Professor Baker needed to write this book, it is necessary to reveal what she herself might be hesitant to tell.

Most people who enter the Arts and Health space fall into one of two categories. We are either artists who grew weary of the soul crushing commoditisation of artistic practice and longed for something more meaningful and edifying of humanity, or health practitioners who grew weary of the objectification of the people in their care and the relentless business drivers that often are at odds with healing, and longed for an approach that did not treat a patient as an item on the assembly line or a community as an aggregate statistic.

Professor Baker is neither of these things. From the age of 15, she knew she wanted to be a music therapist. She intuitively understood the healing power of music and understood also from an early age that intuition was not enough if the practice were ever to be integrated as part of a health system. Professor Baker is not coming to Arts and Health from another field, but from the beginning was a proud practitioner, not unlike a second generation immigrant in a country.

On the one hand, this book is the book she wished someone had written when she was starting out. As it did not exist then, or now, she decided to write it herself. Although ostensibly for Arts and Health professionals, it is a practical guide for any researcher wishing to up their game in terms of scale, relevance, and applicability to real-world implementation and policy.

Yet at the same time, to those who know her, as she is drawing from her own experience and projects of 30 years, it is also a professional autobiography. And with typical modesty (typical for her, not necessarily the field of research), she only could write it down if it served some use to her colleagues and the people she strives to serve.

And in doing so, she has left a lasting testament, edifying the practitioners of Arts and Health around the world, and those they serve.

Which is to say all of us.

Christopher Bailey
Arts and Health Lead
World Health Organization
Geneva, Switzerland

Preface

Over many years, I encountered many academics outside of the creative arts therapies who seemed to have a good grasp of the practicalities of what is needed to implement a good clinical trial. While ideally, my doctoral training should cover that, there are few creative arts therapy researchers that have implemented large trials at any stage in their academic career. There are multiple reasons why this may be the case, none of which are necessary to describe, but nevertheless, there was clearly a whole aspect of training to be a researcher that was missing from my training. As I worked alongside clinician researchers and trialists at both the University of Queensland and University of Melbourne, I learned so much about the complexities of implementing a clinical trial, and soon I found myself being able to write grants that would secure funds to implement them. Over time, I realised that there was a gap in many creative arts therapies researchers' skillset with respect to trial implementation. Hence, the idea of this book was born. I hope it serves its purpose and inspires creative arts therapists to think big and embark on the rewarding journey of leading creative arts therapies trials.

Melbourne, Australia   Felicity Anne Baker

Acknowledgements

There are many people who directly or indirectly have contributed to the contents and thoughts imparted in this book. Firstly, Professor Deborah Theodoros from Speech Pathology at the University of Queensland helped me begin my journey and helped me gain confidence to lead a project, while always mentoring me through it. I acknowledge the long-term contributions of Professor Christian Gold, who I first learned from as we were peers in our doctoral training at Aalborg University Denmark, then went on to collaborate on the MIDDEL project he is leading. We continue to be peers and friends, and I continue to learn from every interaction we have. Through my participation in the MIDDEL, HOME-SIDE, and MATCH projects, I cannot thank enough all my learnings from the incredible mind and most generous and committed researcher Dr. Tanara Sousa. As a health economist, project manager, and just a wonderful human being, I was introduced to the world of REDCap, project and data management, and the notion of setting up systems in place for tracking milestones. Her almost daily probing of tasks that I needed to complete or issues I needed to manage kept me and the project on track. Her input reminded me of the need for strong oversight over every aspect of trial delivery.

When it comes to leading projects, I regularly communicated with Prof. Nicola Lautenschlager, Prof. Helen Odell Miller, and Prof. Karette Stensaeth who would listen to my concerns or issues, and advise on strategies to resolve them. Their endless support, encouragement, and general positivity enabled me to navigate some challenging moments in trial delivery. The incredible HOMESIDE country leaders—Professor Helen Odell Miller, Professor Thomas Wosch, Professor Karette Stensaeth, Dr. Jeanette Tamplin, and Dr. Ania Bukowska—have been invaluable in assisting me in understanding how to coordinate an international trial, one with many moving parts, culturally different ways of working, and ethical challenges concerning local rules. I gained invaluable expertise in managing the many varied challenges in an atmosphere of support and "we-ness" that is necessary for a trial to succeed. My HOMESIDE Australian team—Dr. Jeanette Tamplin, Dr. Libby Flynn, Kate Teggelove, Phoebe Stretton-Smith, Hayley Miller, and Kate McMahon—have helped me gain perspectives on team management and how to be clear about roles, responsibilities, and boundaries. From our MATCH project, working closely with Associate Professors Jenny Waycott, Amit Lampit, Jeanette Tamplin, along with project manager Dr. Tanara Sousa, has provided support while I navigate and learn how to manage a team of more than 30 researchers which spanned the disciplines of clinicians, human computer interaction researchers, software and hardware developers, and trialists [biostatisticians, information scientists, health economists]. Collectively, I needed to pull together a team from disparate disciplines with busy schedules and different levels of commitment to the project. I especially want to thank Associate Professor Amit and Dr. Tanara Sousa for their direct feedback, perspectives on conflicts of interest, and challenging my assumptions about research leadership and team management. They also regularly reminded me that MATCH is my baby and to recognise that not everyone on the team is as invested in the project as me.

I also wish to acknowledge the indirect contributions of several other key people in the University of Melbourne music therapy team, other members of my research teams, the creative arts therapies international alliance and former mentors: Prof. Denise Grocke, Prof. Tony Wigram, Prof. Katrina McFerran, Associate Prof. Grace Thompson, Dr. Imogen Clark, Dr. Lucy Bolger, Associate Prof. Jinah Kim, Prof. Nisha Sajnani, Prof. Vicky Karkou, Prof. Sabine Koch, Prof. Hod Orkibi, and Associate Prof. Becky Zarate.

A special thanks to Christopher Bailey from the World Health Organisation, who has become a recent source of inspiration for me, and now, a friend. Thank you for agreeing to write such a moving Foreword to this book.

Contents

1 **Introduction** 1
Implementing Robust Creative Arts Therapies Trials 1
Sharing Wisdom and Capacity Building 5
So You Won The Grant, Now What? 6
Past and Current Projects 7
   Study 1. Music Therapy to Aid Non-invasive Ventilation Transition for People with Motor Neuron Disease (2014–2015) 8
   Study 2. Singing My Story: Negotiating Identities Through Therapeutic Songwriting for People with Neurological Injuries (2015–2017) 8
   Study 3. MIDDEL: Music Interventions for Dementia and Depression in Elderly Care—The Australian Cohort (2017–2022) 9
   Study 4. HOMESIDE: Home-Based Caregiver Delivered Music Interventions for People Living with Dementia (2019–2022) 10
   Study 5. MATCH: Music Attuned Technology for Care via eHealth (2020–2025) 11
   Study 6. MAPS: Music and Psychology and Social Connections Program (2021–2022) 12
Scope of the Text 12
References 15

2	**The Scope of Project Management**	17
	How Out of Control Can a Controlled Trial Be?	17
	The Project Management Plan	18
	Five Phases of Clinical Trial Project Management	20
	Successful Management Approaches	22
	Good Communication Is Like the Oil in Your Engine	22
	Avoid Meeting Madness	23
	Documentation Avoids Miscommunication	25
	What's Happening Today: Calendar Management	27
	Accountability	28
	Problem Identification and Resolution	28
	Essential Clinical Trial Documents	29
	Study Protocol	30
	Manual of Operational Procedures	32
	Case Report Forms	33
	Clinical Site Management Plan	33
	Risk Management Plan	34
	Developing a Risk Assessment Plan	36
	Types of Risks in Trials	37
	Common Challenges in Clinical Trial Execution	41
	Balancing Complex Workloads	41
	Budget Constraints	42
	Poorly Planned Timelines	43
	Poor Task Prioritisation	43
	Conclusion	44
	References	44
3	**The Art of Good Governance**	47
	What Is Governance?	47
	Governance at Project Design Stage	49
	Governance at Project Authorisation Stage	50
	Governance at Project Implementation Stage and Project Closure	53
	Project Governance Committees	54
	Trial Management Group	54
	Trial Steering Committee	56
	Data Safety Monitoring Board	60
	Project Operational Committees	64
	Whole Team Meetings	64

	Smaller Working Groups and Workstreams	65
	Capacity Building Committee	68
	Statistical Analysis Plan Team	69
	Public and Patient Involvement Committee	70
	Frameworks of PPI	71
	Components of PPI Participation	73
	Reasons the Public Get Involved	75
	Establishing and Implementing a PPI	75
	Conclusion	78
	References	79
4	**Assembling and Uniting a Team**	83
	Staffing to Your Needs	83
	Principal Investigator	88
	Project Manager	90
	Clinical Trial Manager	91
	Biostatistician	92
	Health Economist	93
	Information Scientist	94
	Data Manager	95
	Other Team Members	95
	Optimising Performance: A We-ness Culture	96
	Empowering the Team	97
	Safety Within the Group	98
	Leading the Team	102
	Conclusion	103
	References	103
5	**Budgeting for Success: Management and Resource Planning**	107
	Barriers and Enablers to Effective Resource Management	107
	Preparing a Study Budget	112
	Project Design and Set-Up	112
	Project Implementation	114
	Models to Budget for Recruitment	114
	Licensing Fees	115
	Using Routinely Collected Data	115
	Trial Site Visits and Monitoring	116
	Governance Costs	116
	Data Management and Analysis	116

	Project Management	118
	Public and Patient Involvement and Public Engagement	118
	Knowledge Translation and Exchange, Public Engagement, and Advocacy	118
	Conclusion	119
	References	119
6	**Recruitment, Retention, and Follow-Up: Frustration or Bliss**	121
	Introduction	121
	Why Do People Choose to Participate in Research?	124
	Why Do People Decline Participation in Research?	125
	Health Status and Stigma	125
	Scepticism, Fear and Mistrust	126
	Family Factors	128
	Language Barriers	128
	Participant Burden	129
	Developing and Monitoring the Recruitment Strategy	131
	Participants	132
	Developing the Research Promotional Product	132
	Promoting the Study	134
	Price	137
	Working with Industry Partners	138
	Involvement of Public and Patients in Recruitment	139
	Strategies to Improve Conversion Rates	140
	Harness Trust	140
	Supporting Decision Making	140
	Minimise Burden of Participation	141
	Offering Appropriate Incentives	142
	Working with Your Recruitment Team	142
	Barriers to Participant Retention and Follow-Up	144
	Factors to Increase Retention	145
	Motivating the Recruitment Team	146
	Conclusion	146
	References	146
7	**Quality Data Is Power: Data Management and Monitoring**	151
	The Need for Good Data Management and Monitoring	151
	Defining Quality Data	152

Levels of Data Monitoring	153
The Data Management Plan (DMP)	156
Systems for Data Collection and Management	158
Type of Data and Measures	159
Data Collection Methods	160
Data Entry	162
Data Security	163
Data Cleaning and Quality Control	164
Case Report Forms	169
Data Access: Roles and Responsibilities	169
Data Storage	170
Study Participant Monitoring	172
Data Sharing and Long-Term Preservation	173
Monitoring and Reporting	174
Developing an Electronic Data Capture System for Your Trial	175
Overview of the EDC System Development Process	175
Database User Interface	176
Conclusion	178
References	179

8 Development, Measurement, and Validation of Intervention Fidelity — 183

What Is Fidelity and Why Is It Important?	183
Reporting of Intervention Fidelity in Creative Arts Therapies Literature	186
Conceptual Frameworks of Fidelity	187
Intervention Adherence	187
Assessment of Intervention Components	188
Strategies to Safeguard the Quality of Intervention Delivery	193
Creative Arts Therapist Competence and Training	194
Intervention Supervision and Monitoring	196
Methods of Monitoring Adherence and Exposure	197
Treatment Receipt	201
Treatment Differentiation	203
Treatment Enactment	203
Conclusion	204
References	204

9 Statistical Analysis Plan — 209
What Is a Statistical Analysis Plan? — 209
Why Does a Trial Need a Statistical Analysis Plan? — 209
Developing a Statistical Analysis Plan — 211
Statistical Analysis Plan for Observational Studies — 215
Missing Data — 215
   Approaches to Treat Missing Data — 216
References — 219

10 Development of a Knowledge Translation and Exchange Plan — 223
Our Ethical Responsibility to Disseminate — 223
What Is and Why Implement Knowledge Translation and Exchange? — 224
Dissemination Development Plan — 225
   Research Findings and Products — 225
   Identify End-Users — 228
Collaborating with Partners for Dissemination — 229
Communicating Your Message — 230
Evaluation of Your Dissemination Plan — 231
Strategies and Considerations for Implementing KTE — 232
Authorship and Publishing — 235
Publication Bias — 242
Conclusion — 243
References — 243

11 Innovation, Intellectual Property, and Commercialisation — 247
Innovation — 247
Intellectual Property—Copyright, Patents, Trademarks, and Secrets — 250
Establishing IP Asset Segments — 251
Is Commercialisation a Dirty Word? — 254
Commercialising the Creative Arts Therapies — 255
Engaging with the Business Development Departments at Universities — 257
Assessing Commercial Potential of Your IP — 258
Product Development — 258
   Step 1. Translation of IP into a Proof of Concept — 262

Step 2. Conceptual Design and Development of Low-Fidelity Prototype	265
Step 3. Iterative Design and Evaluation of High-Fidelity Prototype	265
Step 4. Production and Testing of Minimal Viable Product	267
Business Development	268
Competitors	268
Paths to Commercialisation	269
Collaborating with Industry	270
Confidentiality Agreements	272
Establishing a New Arm of Your Team	273
A Word of Caution About Commercialisation	274
Conclusion	274
References	275
Index	**279**

About the Author

Professor Felicity Anne Baker is Associate Dean (Research) at the Faculty of Fine Arts and Music, as well as Director of International Research Partnerships for the Creative Arts and Music Therapy Research Unit, University of Melbourne. She also holds a position as Professor II at the Norwegian Academy of Music and is currently Associate Editor, *Journal of Music Therapy*. Felicity has thirty years of experience as a music therapy clinician and twenty years as a researcher. Over her career, she has accumulated more than AUS$15 million in funding to support implementation of several interdisciplinary clinical trials including three National Health and Medical Research Council Grants and a Medical Research Future Fund grant. She is a former Australia Research Council Future Fellow and has won numerous international awards for her research. She is widely published, and her work is highly cited. Felicity is well known for her research in neurorehabilitation, dementia care, and developing the music therapy method of songwriting. Aside from this latest book, she has published 5 books and more than 170 book chapters and journal articles including publications in *The Lancet Healthy Longevity*, *Contemporary Clinical Trials Communication*, and *Clinical Rehabilitation*.

List of Figures

Fig. 3.1	History of the MATCH project	53
Fig. 3.2	Relationship of working groups to TMG	66
Fig. 6.1	Variability in effectiveness of recruitment strategies of the Australian cohort of the HOMESIDE trial	136
Fig. 7.1	Sample of contour prior to adjustment to frequency levels	166
Fig. 7.2	Results of contour analysis pre-frequency adjustment	167
Fig. 7.3	Sample of contour post adjustment to frequency levels	168
Fig. 7.4	Results of contour analysis post-frequency adjustment	168
Fig. 7.5	HOMESIDE REDCap database home page	177
Fig. 7.6	Example of a HOMESIDE data collection module	178
Fig. 7.7	HOMESIDE Baseline/Follow-ups REDCap Dashboard	179
Fig. 9.1	Excerpt from HOMESIDE Statistical Analysis Plan	219
Fig. 11.1	Examples of MATCH trademarked logo	252
Fig. 11.2	Technology development timeline	263
Fig. 11.3	Example of initial wireframes of MATCH	266
Fig. 11.4	(**a**) Layers of collaborators. (**b**) Layers of collaborators in MATCH	271

List of Tables

Table 2.1	Risk action plan for the Australian MIDDEL recruitment strategy	38
Table 2.2	HOMESIDE home visit risk assessment	40
Table 7.1	Contents of a Data Management Plan	157
Table 7.2	HOMESIDE REDCap Roles	171
Table 8.1	Music intervention caregiver training fidelity checklist—training session 1	191
Table 8.2	Treatment receipt examples in creative arts therapy research	202
Table 11.1	Assessment of commercial potential of MATCH	259

CHAPTER 1

Introduction

Implementing Robust Creative Arts Therapies Trials

When I started out as a music therapy researcher back in 1997, creative arts therapies research was predominantly conducted on a small scale. Published studies with sample sizes greater than 50 were rare, and almost entirely published in the *Journal of Music Therapy* and absent from any interdisciplinary health journal. A scope of the publications from *Arts in Psychotherapy* and *International Journal of Art Therapy* highlights a similar picture. We as creative arts therapy researchers strive to advocate for different forms of "evidence" and believe that studies of lived experience and consumer perspectives are critical to advancing understanding of our research impact. Indeed, these discipline specialist journals are a good forum for documenting such outcomes. Several countries have made progress in the recognition of the "evidence" lived experience-based research provides. However, on a global scale, there is still some way to go to arrive at a point where all forms of evidence are recognised as "equal".

The "medical models of research" still dominate the healthcare sector and subsequently the research funding outcomes, and, if we want to play with the big players, we do at times have to try to accommodate their approaches to research and create the types of quality evidence that lead to recognition, credibility, visibility, and acceptability. For a long while, I struggled with navigating the tension within me. I was frustrated (and remain so at times) with the expectation to conform to research paradigms and practices that at face value seemed to be odds with the very nature of creative arts therapies. The "controlled" nature of a randomised controlled trial seems incongruent with the aims of the creative arts therapies where we create therapeutic conditions that promote and value free expression at the individual level rather than at a population level. Everyone's experiences are equally valued, and in essence their own individual evidence of the impact of creative arts therapies on their wellbeing. But it is unlikely that small-scale studies of lived experience will be regarded as high impact and reach the pages of medical journals such as *The Lancet*, *New England Journal of Medicine*, *Journal of the American Medical Association*, or *British Medical Journal*. Publications in such journals are often accompanied by public facing media releases which can be mechanisms for advocacy. These then allow spaces for telling the individual stories of participants and what their participation in creative arts therapies meant for them. Similarly, articles in the aforementioned prestigious journals create opportunities for raising awareness of the evidence with key stakeholders and people responsible for shaping policies.

I have more recently addressed my internal tension around what is "evidence" and have had lively debates with many colleagues about this over the last years. Since being a founding member of the International Research Alliance for the Creative Arts Therapies (https://steinhardt.nyu.edu/catconsortium/international-research-alliance), I discovered that elsewhere around the world and within the other creative arts therapies disciplines (dance/movement, art, drama, psychodrama, poetry), similar tensions were being experienced. I came to understand that it did not need to be an either/or scenario but that smaller-scale interpretivist projects could be forms of evidence nested within a larger randomised controlled trial. I do not regard these as mixed methods studies, but more there are sub-studies within a larger project. An excellent example of this is within our project HOMESIDE which I describe in more detail later in this chapter. Within a larger randomised controlled trial, HOMESIDE had several sub-projects that were focused on analysing the extensive qualitative data we had collected from interviews, participant diaries, and fortnightly phone calls. Over the course of HOMESIDE, we enrolled seven doctoral students (3 in the United Kingdom, and one each in Australia, Poland, Norway and Germany), and each student carved out their own sub-project. These sub-projects could focus in on the nuances of the intervention and participant responses that are not captured in the quantitative findings. Similarly, we established five research teams to explore participants' lived experiences as well as identify patterns in the data that could help us refine the intervention.

But let me return to the discussion point of why there may be very few creative arts therapies studies that are published in the high-impact interdisciplinary journals. One must first ask, what types of studies "make it in"? When I surveyed a few of my colleagues about their thoughts, and reviewed the few studies that were published, several common themes arose. First, these journals have a success rate of about 5% and therefore only accept the top 5% submitted. A triage system is usually in place whereby one of the associate editors reviews the manuscript to assess whether it meets the criteria for publication in their journal. Many journals require manuscripts have clear and powerful statements of what is the added value of the study, and whether the study is robust enough and sufficiently powered to justify the claims the findings make. While small-scale projects that are underpowered are important to our fields, they usually have little policy-changing influences and therefore are not of interest to high-impact journals.

Another obvious reason why studies are not robust relates to research funding. Large-scale fully powered clinical trials cost money, a lot of money. Multiple team members are needed to ensure randomisation processes are well designed, data collected is of high quality and by team members who are masked to condition, and interventions are protocolised and fidelity assessed. Many of these trial management processes are described in this book. If there is insufficient funding to implement the trial, it may be near impossible to deliver a high-quality non-biased study.

Finally, many proposed studies cannot attract funding or if they are completed are not published in the most prestigious journals, because they present with too many methodological flaws due to inexperience or the lack of training of creative arts therapies researchers. And while I still learn everyday as new research practices continue to evolve, I definitely regarded myself as being in the category of an "under" trained researcher until I recognised that and sought to develop my skills. Evidence of the absence of robust studies in the creative arts therapies fields is found in the quality appraisal of studies contained in systematic reviews. For example, in a systematic review of creative arts therapies studies focused on addressing post-traumatic stress disorder, all included studies were assessed as low to very low in quality (Baker et al., 2018). Similar outcomes were evident in a review of studies addressing depression in older adults (Dunphy et al., 2019) as well as in review studies of the individual creative arts therapy disciplines across a range of clinical populations (e.g. Feniger-Schaal & Orkibi, 2020; Golubovic et al., 2022; Karkou et al., 2019). Therefore, the potential for these reviews to be used to influence policy and inform changes to practice is limited.

The question remains as to why creative arts therapy researchers are not designing robust studies. Why are we not receiving the rigorous training in trial designs that many of our counterparts are in the other health science disciplines?[1] In my view, this scenario is the result of two interrelated issues, all stemming from the fact that most creative arts therapies university programs are located within fine and performing arts faculties, conservatories, or in the humanities faculties. First, it is usual practice that to be competitive for large-scale funding needed to implement the fully powered studies, feasibility and pilot studies are needed. Inevitably, these smaller studies also require adequate resourcing. If the creative arts therapies researchers are located within a humanities or creative arts faculty, it is highly likely that their Faculty Dean (or equivalent title dependent upon university structures) may be a creative arts performer, artist, historian, or a philosopher who is often not accustomed to the unique research needs and activities those in the creative arts therapies. Many other disciplines within these faculties work as individuals on their own archival or artistic research. Trying to illustrate to a dean that a US$20,000 university-funded internal grant will not go far even in a small feasibility study is challenging, when the majority of researchers within the faculty could make $5,000 go a long way. Without access to sufficient funding for a feasibility study, the opportunity to access external funding to implement is near impossible.

In addition to limited access to university internal funding, because creative arts therapists are often located in these fine and performing arts or humanities faculties, many may not have access to collaborate with and learn from researchers from other health disciplines. When I felt sufficiently confident to develop and trial high-impact research and design

---

[1] I would like to add here that I am definitely not suggesting that all creative arts therapy researchers have not received rigorous training in trial design, but many have not. This trend, however, is changing as a growing group of creative arts therapy researchers from a select number of universities are being better trained and consequently passing on their skills and knowledge to the next generation. For example, the researchers belong to the Universities from the International Research Alliance of Creative Arts Therapies (https://steinhardt.nyu.edu/catconsortium/international-research-alliance).

a fully powered study, it was through my interaction with researchers located in our Faculty of Medicine, Dentistry, and Health Science that I came to realise the true value of interdisciplinary research teams and insight into how much I really did not know about implementing a trial. So, while my music therapy colleagues have been invaluable in helping me to deepen and expand perspectives about music therapy research, I began to realise that I needed to seek expertise outside of my discipline to gain the skills and knowledge that I have now. That's not to say I know everything. Not at all. I'm still learning, and the research landscape keeps evolving. Every time I am introduced to a new researcher from a new field, I learn and integrate that learning into my own research plans and management approaches. For example, at the time of writing this book, I just begun the MATCH project (see later this chapter), which comprised of a team of 20 investigators spanning 13 different health disciplines. One such researcher Dr Amit Lampit, a cognitive neuroscientist, was recruited to our team to lead one of the workstreams. Through our co-supervision of a doctoral student, I was introduced to the notion of network meta-analysis and component network meta-analysis.[2]

SHARING WISDOM AND CAPACITY BUILDING

As I gained this somewhat incidentally acquired knowledge over my 20+ years of engaging in research, I have been committed to sharing my learnings, experiences, and wisdom with other creative arts therapy researchers. The notion of capacity building—the process of developing and strengthening the skills, instincts, abilities, processes, and resources that organisations and communities need to survive, adapt, and thrive in a fast-changing world (United Nations, n.d.)—is something I am passionate about, and I consider necessary for our disciplines to grow and flourish. The types of knowledge and expertise I have gained as a research leader (principal investigator) go beyond what is possible to learn within a creative arts therapies doctoral training program; these are skills

---

[2] Network meta-analysis is a technique for comparing three or more interventions simultaneously in a single analysis by combining both direct evidence and indirect evidence across a network of studies. It produces estimates of the relative effects between any pair of interventions in the network, and usually yields more precise estimates than a single direct or indirect estimate (Chaimani et al., 2022). A component network meta-analysis extends this further. It takes the studies where interventions may have multiple components and seeks to analyse the impact of each component (Rücker et al., 2020).

that even mid-career researchers 10-years post-PhD may not yet have had an opportunity to learn or experience. One of the main explanations for a lack of knowledge about how to implement trials is that our creative arts therapies disciplines have had a tradition of encouraging prospective doctoral candidates to develop and implement their own independent projects. While this tradition of a stand-alone study is changing, it remains the dominant approach to doctoral training. This tradition is distinctly different to the traditions in other health disciplines where the doctoral projects that candidates engage in are often nested within a larger project. These doctoral candidates have the benefit of being involved in an interdisciplinary team, have access to broad expertise, and receive mentoring and exposure to how large clinical trials are led and managed right from the outset. There is certainly truth in the saying that researchers don't know what they don't know. From my own experience, my awareness and learnings often occurred from interacting with other researchers outside of my discipline.

Having doctoral candidates learn through their participation in a larger project was something I aspired to adopt if given an opportunity to. And this opportunity emerged when the international HOMESIDE team secured funding to implement a large randomised controlled trial across 5 countries. Within our trial, 7 doctoral candidates and 6 postdoctoral research fellows worked alongside biostatisticians, psychiatrists, health economists, database managers, and information scientists and had support from 12 chief investigators. This was the type of doctoral and post-doctoral training I never had but would have clearly benefited from.

So You Won The Grant, Now What?

The main purpose of this book is to provide support and guidance in project management and implementation for those researchers embarking on this monumental challenge. Securing the funds to support the project is just the key to opening the gate, one must walk through it and use the money wisely and in a planned and monitored manner to ensure that the project does not lead to research waste.[3] An ethical movement by researchers to reduce and avoid research waste is gaining momentum at present that (Gardener, 2018), with the argument that "we need

---

[3] Research waste is a term commonly used to describe the poor use of money and resources that have led to no useful outcomes.

less research, better research, and research done for the right reasons" (Altman, 1994).

Throughout this text, I outline the various study implementation components and influencing factors that can directly or indirectly impact project success.[4] Each chapter offers guidance ranging from considering the composition of your research team, registering your trial before you enrol your first participant, planning your recruitment strategy at the time of developing your budgets, and identifying a list of project risks and strategies to mitigate them. These types of leadership and management considerations are not typically described in other texts about research methodology. There are literally hundreds of research method books in the health sciences, and a handful focused on the creative arts therapies (e.g. McFerran & Silverman, 2018; Wheeler & Murphy, 2016), that describe everything from formulating your research question, analysis of qualitative data, research designs, to research ethics, but none provide guidance in implementation. This book aims to fill this gap, to guide the researcher starting from the point when the project proposal has been finalised and then walks the novice research leader through practical post-design implementation considerations. It aims to equip researchers with knowledge that will help them plan for implementation and to be cognisant of the potential pitfalls associated with leading a team of researchers. In imparting my own knowledge and wisdom, I provide real-world accounts of my own experiences, highlighting when things went right and wrong, and what I learned from them. By breaking down the components of the clinical trial landscape and stepping the researcher through the clinical implementation trial journey, I hope you the reader will have a deeper understanding of the research process at scale and a reduced level of anxiety about scaling up your research to a size where it can have policy-changing impact.

Past and Current Projects

Within each chapter of this book, I describe real-world examples of how I navigated challenges associated with leading a project and a project team. While the examples will be drawn from projects dating back to my first

---

[4] The term project success is an interesting philosophical question. What does success mean? What does it look like? For me, success is the completion of a study that has been executed with rigor and care, and whereby the findings can be trusted—even when those findings tell a different narrative to that expected or hoped for.

study in 1997, most experiences I report on occurred during the implementation of the more recent and larger studies involving interdisciplinary teams. As I will be referring to them frequently, it is important that I briefly summarise them in chronological order as I will not be describing them in each chapter but rather providing links back to their descriptions here.

Study 1. Music Therapy to Aid Non-invasive Ventilation Transition for People with Motor Neuron Disease (2014–2015)

This feasibility study of a music intervention to support non-invasive ventilation (NIV) transition for people with Motor Neuron Disease (MND, also referred to as Amyotrophic lateral sclerosis) was a unique collaboration between the University of Melbourne, Victorian Respiratory Support Service (Austin Health) and Calvary Healthcare Bethlehem. This project, for the first time, explored the use of an individually designed music and relaxation program that people with MND could use to aid their NIV transition (Tamplin et al., 2017). The study involved music therapy researchers, music therapy clinicians, as well as experts in respiratory medicine and respiratory physiotherapy. The feasibility study allowed participants to self-select into their chosen group—with music assisted support or without it. Data on NIV use was collected directly from the Continuous Positive Airway Pressure in the first 7-days post-baseline to determine adherence to NIV use. We also collected data about music use to determine whether music increases adherence to NIV use. Participants reported its value in distracting and relaxing them while using NIV but quantitative data was inconclusive.

Study 2. Singing My Story: Negotiating Identities Through Therapeutic Songwriting for People with Neurological Injuries (2015–2017)

This interdisciplinary project funded by the Australian Research Council Discovery Project (DP150100201) was a pilot randomised controlled trial that examined the use of therapeutic songwriting on the transformation of identity of people with brain injury or spinal cord injury who were either in-patients involved in active rehabilitation or who had been living in the community 2+ years post-discharge (Baker, Tamplin, Rickard, et al., 2019). Participants created 3 songs using a purposefully designed intervention protocol over 12 sessions using established domains of identity to inform the intervention design (Tamplin et al., 2016). We adopted several standardised measures to determine changes in self-concept, satisfaction with life, depression, and emotion regulation. As expected, due to the small sample size ($n = 47$), no significant between group pre–post intervention differences were found on the primary self-concept measure; however, the size of the effects (Songwriting group: $d = 0.44$; standard care $d = 0.08$) suggested that a fully powered trial was warranted. We also found that there were significant and large effect sizes from baseline to post between groups in favour of the songwriting group for Satisfaction with Life. Emotion regulation improved in the group receiving songwriting but again due to the small sample size was not statistically significant. We found that the songwriting intervention was also more acceptable and feasible for use with community-dwelling people rather than in-patients involved in active rehabilitation programs.

Study 3. MIDDEL: Music Interventions for Dementia and Depression in Elderly Care—The Australian Cohort (2017–2022)

Funded by Australia's National Health and Medical Research Council (GNT1137853), this project was a cluster randomised controlled trial that compared group music therapy, recreational choir singing, both and neither (four arms) on the depression (primary) and neuropsychiatric symptoms, quality of life, and costs of people with dementia living in residential aged care homes over a 12-month period (Baker et al., 2022). This project was part of a larger trial led by Professor Christian Gold involving Norway, Germany, United Kingdom, Turkey, and the Netherlands (JPND2019-466-067 [https://www.middel-project.eu/]). However, Australia was successful at securing funding first and had completed collecting its data before the other countries had even commenced. This trial was significantly interrupted by COVID-19 lockdowns; nevertheless, we collected data on 318 participants of our target 500. We recruited 24 care home units (24 clusters), but only 20 were included due to the COVID-19 pandemic. Disciplines involved in this study included music therapists, geriatricians, biostatisticians, information scientists, and health economists.

As described in Chapter 8, we designed and implemented a fidelity protocol (Baker, Tamplin, Clark, et al., 2019), which was used in the larger international study. We also undertook an analysis of resource use around recruitment and assessment of outcome measures (Baker et al., 2020). Understanding the time and effort required to recruit and assess is important for clinical trials as it speaks to the feasibility of the study, the estimated timeframe to collect data and to costing the study. I discuss this at length in Chapter 5. For example, we found that the time between initially contacting next of kin to determine whether they gave permission for their loved one to participate, to actually receiving formal consent, often exceeded 45 days. We also calculated the ratio of time between direct and indirect research activity when our assessors were on site at residential aged care homes and found that for every one hour of data collection, another two hours was spent there waiting for residents to be available or waiting for staff assistance. Despite COVID-19 lockdowns and associated deaths, we found significant findings on our primary outcome measure of depression suggesting beneficial effects of recreational choir singing, but not group music therapy (Baker et al., 2022).

Study 4. HOMESIDE: Home-Based Caregiver Delivered Music Interventions for People Living with Dementia (2019–2022)

HOMESIDE (https://www.homesidestudy.eu/) is an international randomised controlled trial that, like MIDDEL, was also funded through the Joint Programme for Neurodegenerative Diseases. Countries involved in this study were Australia, Norway, Germany, Poland, and the United Kingdom. The trial tested the effectiveness of a family caregiver delivered music intervention on the neuropsychiatric symptoms (primary), depression, quality of life, and costs of the person living with dementia, as well as on wellbeing outcomes for the caregiver (Baker, Bloska, et al., 2019). In this trial, family caregivers participated in three music intervention training sessions that aimed to provide them with tools to use music in a more intentional way to support the care of their family member with dementia at home. They were then expected to use these skills to engage their loved one in music experiences at least twice per week for 12 weeks. This randomised controlled trial compared the music intervention with a comparative reading condition and standard care. The diversity of disciplines within the team included music therapists, occupational therapists, old age psychiatrists, data managers, biostatisticians, and health economists. Each country had its own team of researchers, post-doctoral researchers, and doctoral candidates. At the time of writing this book, the project was at the tail end of collecting data and findings are expected to be published in the latter half of 2023.

Study 5. MATCH: Music Attuned Technology for Care via eHealth (2020–2025)

Funded for AUS$2 million by Australia's Medical Research Future Fund (MRFF2007411), MATCH (https://www.musicattunedcare.com/) is an eHealth development and feasibility study focused on translating the HOMESIDE in-person training into a digitally delivered training program. In addition, MATCH has artificial intelligence embedded into it to (a) detect a change in agitation based on wearable devices and environmental sensors that detect changes in movement patterns and speech patterns, (b) select music that appropriately matches the level of agitation, and (c) then continuously adapts the music to attune to and regulate the person living with dementia. Building on HOMESIDE, this project aims to also embed a professional caregiver training program for staff caring for people living in residential aged care homes and it will also explore the use in transitional contexts (when people move from home into residential aged care). The project has four streams: (1) translation of music therapy into digital content, (2) co-designing the app features with end-users, (3) software and hardware development to develop the machine learning and artificial intelligence features, and (4) the clinical team who implement and test this in the field. This project is the most interdisciplinary project I have ever been involved in which includes 20 investigators (in addition to post-doctoral researchers and project team members) from music therapy, speech pathology, physiotherapy, psychiatry, neuropsychology, health education, hardware and software engineering, digital health, human computer interaction, health economy, and biostatistics. The project began in 2020 when we received more than AUS$100,000 from University of Melbourne alumni to begin the project. In 2021, we received an additional $100,000 from the University's Proof of Concept fund. During those two years, we developed and co-designed the first version of the mobile application which comprised entirely of the family caregiver training program. The additional artificial intelligence features were not yet being developed.

Study 6. MAPS: Music and Psychology and Social Connections Program (2021–2022)

MAPS is a collaboration between neuropsychiatry, psychology, and music therapy and is being led by neuropsychiatrist Dr Samantha Loi (Loi et al., 2022). In this study, therapeutic songwriting, cognitive behaviour therapy, and a private social networking group form an interdisciplinary intervention designed to support people with young onset dementia and their care partners. The intervention was informed by a theory of adaptive coping specifically focused on dyads affected by young onset dementia (Bannon et al., 2021). In the first instance, we are implementing a randomised controlled trial with a waitlist control. The primary aims are to assess whether our intervention improves depressive, anxiety, and stress symptoms in caregivers, with secondary aims to assess whether the intervention improves depressive symptoms in people with young onset dementia. Our 60 dyads will participate in a group-based weekly online program for 8 weeks facilitated by a music therapist and psychologist. Sessions 1 and 8 will include both caregivers and people with young onset dementia while Sessions 2–7 will involve separate group sessions for caregivers and those with dementia.

SCOPE OF THE TEXT

My hope in publishing this book is that many early and mid-career researchers can benefit from the discoveries, failures, and learnings I have encountered over the past 20+ years thereby enabling them to design and implement successful impactful research. As already mentioned, this is not a research methods book, but a book about study implementation. While my experience is in music therapy, I assert that the learnings are translatable to all creative arts therapies. Wherever possible, I have tried to incorporate studies of my peers in dance/movement therapy, drama therapy, and psychodrama and art therapy and have consulted with them to ensure this text is appropriate and relevant for those disciplines too.

The structure of the content and its organisation are intentionally very digestible. As researchers, we are often reading complex texts as part of our day-to-day life. Therefore, I aimed to minimise any additional burden by writing chapters that were accessible and deliberately effortless to read. For the most part, the chapters are theory-free, purposefully informal in style, and are highly practical. Intermittently, I offer reflections on my decisions and actions, especially when they led to counterproductive outcomes. Wherever possible, I propose alternative actions.

This text is divided into 11 chapters. This chapter introduces the reader to the whole text and briefly describes the main studies that informed this book and that are referred to throughout the remaining chapters. Chapter 2 introduces the reader to the concept of clinical trial project management. I begin with describing the five phases of clinical trial management—initiation, planning, execution, monitoring, and closing—as these set the scene for the remaining chapters. The chapter then provides reflections on successful management approaches including team communication, accountability, problem identification and resolution, and the creation of efficient systems. Approaches to risk management are included as the principal investigator is accountable for implementing a safe and successful trial. Later in the chapter, I detail various clinical trial management tools that can help the principal investigator to adhere to the project timeline. The essential trial documents are described including the study protocol, trial registration, and the standard operating procedures (project manual). The chapter concludes with some of the common challenges in clinical trial execution that I have encountered.

Chapter 3 provides an overview of the governance requirements needed to ensure trials are of high quality, rigorous, safe, and will finish on time, on budget, and with an excellent high-quality data set. The chapter describes the role of governance at different points in the trial and the objectives of each type of trial committee. The chapter concludes with an overview of the role and operations of the public and patient involvement committee. The assemblance, uniting, and leadership of an interdisciplinary team are the focus of Chapter 4. I explain the various roles of the trial team and what to consider in ensuring you to get the right mix of skills. Later in the chapter, I focus on the importance of creating a "we-ness" and how to get the best out of your team by recognising how different personalities—action-oriented, people-oriented, and thinking-oriented—can benefit the project.

In Chapter 5, I provide guidance in how to prepare and monitor an accurate trial budget. I outline the many trial-related costs that researchers need to consider when preparing trial budgets and reflect on my own experience of what aspects of clinical trial implementation were more resource intensive. In the final section of the trial, there are clear descriptions of how to plan a budget for the different components of the trial—project design and set-up; ethics, contracts, and other regulatory processes; monitoring and quality assurance; trial master file handling and administration; data management; statistics, report, and publication; project management; patient and public involvement; and site costs.

One of the most challenging aspects of any large clinical trial is participant recruitment. In Chapter 6, I provide an overview of issues related to successful or unsuccessful recruitment strategies including a review of why people choose or decline participation. Barriers to recruitment such as mistrust of researchers, stigma around diagnosis, language, psychological, physical or financial burden, and gatekeeper concerns are outlined. The chapter then describes various approaches to recruit participants in particular understanding the "market", developing appropriate promotional materials, and releasing and assessing the impact of these within the market. Finally, the chapter includes considerations around participant retention and follow-up and motivating the team to sustain recruitment efforts.

Data management and monitoring is the focus of Chapter 7. It describes the considerations for and importance of a comprehensive database to minimise the risk of collecting low quality, inaccurate, incomplete, or missing data. The chapter outlines the components of a data management plan including the types of data being collected, the data collection methods to capture the data, processes to safeguard data quality including data entry, security, and cleaning. The chapter includes descriptions of how to design an electronic data capturing system and how these systems can be utilised for controlling data access, increasing the reliability and completeness of the data set, and enabling efficient data reporting. In Chapter 8, I present an overview of the concept of fidelity and how to develop measurement tools and validation processes to strengthen the reliability and validity of the study.

Chapter 9 outlines the process of developing a statistical analysis plan and the key components of one. While the plan is initiated and led by the biostatistical team, the principal investigator and other key members of the research team do need to input into it so a thorough understanding of its role and process in the trial is needed. Devising a carefully considered and relevant dissemination and knowledge translation plan is important; otherwise, the research does not achieve its primary aim—to improve the health and wellbeing of a population. In Chapter 10, I outline how to develop such a plan to ensure that a wide variety of audiences are reached. I also offer some guidance on negotiating authorship, something that becomes a sensitive issue as the team grows. Finally, Chapter 11 completes this text by focusing on aspects of innovation, intellectual property, and commercialisation of the research.

References

Altman, D. G. (1994). The scandal of poor medical research. *British Medical Journal, 308*(6924), 283–284.

Baker, F. A., Bloska, J., Stensæth, K., Wosch, T., Bukowska, A., Braat, S., Sousa, T., Tamplin, J., Clark, I. N., Lee, Y.-E. C., Clarke, P., Lautenschlager, N., & Odell-Miller, H. (2019). HOMESIDE: A home-based family caregiver-delivered music intervention for people living with dementia: Protocol of a randomised controlled trial. *British Medical Journal Open*. https://doi.org/10.1136/bmjopen-2019-031332

Baker, F. A., Lee, Y.-E. C., Sousa, T. V., Stretton-Smith, P. A., Tamplin, J., Sveinsdottir, V., Geretsegger, M., Wake, J. D., Assmus, J., & Christian Gold, C. (2022). Clinical effectiveness of Music Interventions for Dementia and Depression in Elderly care [MIDDEL] in the Australian cohort: Pragmatic cluster-randomised controlled trial. *The Lancet Healthy Longevity, 3*(3), e153–e165.

Baker, F. A., Metcalf, O., Varker, T., & O'Donnell, M. (2018, November). A systematic review of the efficacy of creative arts therapies in the treatment of adults with PTSD. *Psychological Trauma: Theory, Research, Practice, and Policy, 10*(6), 643–651. http://dx.doi.org/10.1037/tra0000353

Baker, F. A., Stretton-Smith, P., Sousa, T. A., Clark, I., Cotton, A., Gold, C., & Lee, Y.-E. C. (2020). Process and resource assessment in trials undertaken in residential care homes: Experiences from the Australian MIDDEL research team. *Contemporary Clinical Trials Communication*. https://doi.org/10.1016/j.conctc.2020.100675

Baker, F. A., Tamplin, J., Clark, I., Lee, Y.-E. C., Geretsegger, M., & Gold, C. (2019). Treatment fidelity in a music therapy multi-site cluster randomized control trial for people living with dementia: The MIDDEL project. *Journal of Music Therapy*. https://doi.org/10.1093/jmt/thy023

Baker, F. A., Tamplin, J., Rickard, N., Ponsford, J., New, P., & Lee, Y.-E. C. (2019). A therapeutic songwriting intervention to promote reconstruction of self-concept and enhance wellbeing following brain and spinal cord injury: Pilot randomised controlled trial. *Clinical Rehabilitation*. https://doi.org/10.1177/0123456789123456. First Published 22 February 2019.

Bannon, S. M., Reichman, M., Popok, P., Grunberg, V. A., Traeger, L., Gates, M. V., Krahn, E. A., Brandt, K., Quimby, M., Wong, B., Dickerson, B. C. & Vranceanu, A.-M. (2021). Psychosocial stressors and adaptive coping strategies in couples after a diagnosis of Young-Onset Dementia. *The Gerontologist, 62*, 262–275.

Chaimani, A., Caldwell, D. M., Li, T., Higgins, J. P. T., & Salanti, G. (2022). Undertaking network meta-analyses. In J. P. T. Higgins, J. Thomas, J. Chandler, M. Cumpston, T. Li, M. J. Page, & V. A. Welch (Eds.), *Cochrane handbook for systematic reviews of interventions* (Version 6.3). www.training.cochrane.org/handbook

Dunphy, K., Baker, F. A., Dumaresq, E., Carroll-Haskins, K., Eickholt, J., Ercole, M., Kaimal, G., Meyer, K., Sajnani, N., Shamir, O. Y., & Wosch, T. (2019). Creative arts interventions to address depression in older adults: A systematic review of outcomes, processes, and mechanisms. *Frontiers in Psychology, 9*, 2655. https://doi.org/10.3389/fpsyg.2018.02655

Feniger-Schaal, R., & Orkibi, H. (2020). Integrative systematic review of drama therapy intervention research. *Psychology of Aesthetics, Creativity & the Arts, 14*(1), 68–80.

Gardener, H. (2018). *Making clinical trials more efficient: Consolidating, communicating and improving knowledge of participant recruitment interventions.* PhD Thesis. University of Aberdeen, Scotland.

Golubovic, J., Neerland, B. E., & Baker, F. A. (2022). Music interventions and management of delirium in adults: A systematic review and meta-analysis. *Brain Sciences, 12*, 568. https://doi.org/10.3390/brainsci12050568

Karkou, K., Aithal, S., Zubala, A., & Meekums, B. (2019). Effectiveness of dance movement therapy in the treatment of adults with depression: A systematic review with meta-analyses. *Frontiers in Psychology*, 10. https://doi.org/doi.org/10.3389/fpsyg.2019.00936

Loi, S. M., Flynn, L., Cadwallader, C., Stretton-Smith, P., Bryant, C., & Baker, F. A. (2022). Music and psychology & social connections program: Protocol for a novel intervention for dyads affected by Younger-Onset Dementia. *Brain Sciences, 12*, 503. https://doi.org/10.3390/brainsci12040503

McFerran, K., & Silverman, M. J. (2018). *A guide to designing research questions for beginning music therapy researchers.* American Music Therapy Association.

Rücker, G., Petropoulou, M., & Schwarzer, G. (2020). Network meta-analysis of multicomponent interventions. *Biometrical Journal, 62*(3), 808–821. https://doi.org/10.1002/bimj.201800167

Tamplin, J., Baker, F. A., Bolger, K., Bajo, E., Davies, R., Sheers, N., & Berlowitz, D. (2017). Exploring the feasibility of music-assisted relaxation intervention on the transition to non-invasive ventilation in people with Motor Neuron Disease. *Music Medicine, 19*(2), 86–97.

Tamplin, J., Baker, F. A., Rickard, N., Roddy, C., & MacDonald, R. (2016). A theoretical framework and therapeutic songwriting protocol to promote integration of self-concept in people with acquired neurological injuries. *Nordic Journal of Music Therapy, 25*(2), 111–133. https://doi.org/10.1080/08098131.2015.1011208

United Nations. (n.d.). *Capacity building.* https://www.un.org/en/academic-impact/capacity-building. Accessed 30 July 2022.

Wheeler, B. L., & Murphy, K. M. (2016). *Music therapy research.* Barcelona Publishers.

CHAPTER 2

The Scope of Project Management

How Out of Control Can a Controlled Trial Be?

Managing clinical trials, of whatever size and complexity, demands that the principal investigator[1] together with the project manager[2] implements planned and efficient trial management processes. I know from first-hand experience that there are many moving parts to a trial, interdependencies between components, that it can quickly feel like the controlled trial is out of control. Having spoken with many colleagues, I know this experience is not unique. Good management and governance are needed to keep the trial under control. Indeed, the Medical Research Council (2003) indicated that many trials were not successful due to management issues rather than weaknesses in the trial design. Farrell et al. (2010) intimated that many trials fail to achieve their aims because there was a lack of structured, practical, business-like approaches to management. While well-designed trials are needed to answer the clinical questions posed, the science alone is not the key to success. Management of time, money,

---

[1] Dependent upon local traditions, the term principal investigator, chief investigator, and lead investigator have been used interchangeably to describe the investigator who leads the research team. In this book, I choose to use the term principal investigator to indicate the lead researcher and the term chief investigator to indicate a researcher who is listed on the grant and has specific responsibilities to lead a "component" of the project.

[2] The project manager coordinates the daily operations of the trial in consultation with the principal investigator.

and staffing is needed to ensure the trial delivers within the expected timeframe and to budget.

Historically, knowledge about trial management systems and implementation has typically been passed down through apprenticeship or mentorship models rather than by formalised training. This has been true of my experiences to date. I learned all I could from my doctoral supervisor the late and great Professor Tony Wigram, and now the additional knowledge I have acquired is passed down to my doctoral students and post-doctoral fellows. Sadly, knowledge about trial implementation and management has not been documented, evaluated, or published (Farrell et al., 2010). The flow on effect is that researchers have "invented and reinvented the trial management wheel" (Farrell et al., 2010).

The Project Management Plan

Developing a project management plan is the first step to avoiding a controlled trial becoming out of control. It's the first major task that the principal investigator and project manager must prepare. The more detailed the plan is, the more efficiently and accurately the project can be tracked and monitored. At the same time, the project management plan should be considered a living document. Without a sense of direction, it can be easy to feel overwhelmed, unsure of what tasks need to be undertaken, and when, and by whom. The plan allows for a clear direction, documents timelines and milestones, and creates a plan for who within the team is responsible for different aspects of the project.

In the context of a creative arts therapies clinical trial, a project management plan is "dynamic set of documents" (ISAC & IFAR, 2018) that clearly outlines the goals and provides roadmap for the project. Included in the plan are details of the deliverables, the tasks, timelines, and resources (personnel and direct costs) needed to achieve those deliverables and processes that will ensure they are achieved according to the highest quality standards. Ultimately, the plan is designed to help the team organise their activities, manage the various tasks (and the interdependencies between tasks), ensure transparency of processes and those responsible for undertaking them, and monitor and detect early, any issues that may threaten the successful completion of the project. Importantly, the plan guides the research team to ensure the project moves forward according to the timeline, so it can meet planned key performances indicators, milestones, and deliverables.

While a detailed plan is critical, the plan is not necessarily fixed and unchanging, but can be agile and adaptable. As the project unfolds, unexpected enablers or barriers to implementation present themselves, which point to the need for project planning adaptation. Two excellent examples of changing a plan were evident in both the MIDDEL (Baker et al., 2022) and HOMESIDE (Baker et al., 2019) projects as they had to adapt to unforeseeable external factors caused by the COVID-19 pandemic (see project descriptions in Chapter 1). In the MIDDEL residential age music interventions project, many care homes were in COVID-enforced locked down for extended periods; some for more than 12 months. These lockdowns meant that our assessors collecting data and our music group facilitators were able to be present on site to undertake their tasks. Part of our response to the pandemic was that we explored remote delivery of interventions. However, three of the four treatment arms utilised group singing as a key activity. At the time, singing was regarded as a high COVID-19 transmission risk and consequently, all interventions ceased. While not ideal, we adapted our assessment processes by administering them over the phone with care home staff so that we could retain as many of the enrolled participants as possible. As the lockdowns continued in Melbourne, the Data Safety Monitoring Board (Chapter 3), in conjunction with the principal investigator, made the call to cease recruitment with just 64% of our target sample randomised and receiving all or a portion of the intervention. We revised our plans according to these external uncontrollable factors.

In our international HOMESIDE project being implemented in Australia, Germany, Norway, Poland, and the United Kingdom, we were testing the effectiveness of family carers of people with dementia to use music mindfully to support care. The intervention involved music therapists visiting the participants three times to provide training in the intentional use of music. However, the emergence of COVID-19 also led us to adapt our project plan as visits to participants' homes were no longer permitted. In this study, we had only recruited 19 of our 495 participant dyads (people living with dementia and their carers), and after consultation with our Data Safety Monitoring Board, we adapted the study protocol so that music training sessions were implemented online, and data was collected remotely. While we were adamant that our music training would be more effective if delivered face to face, the advantage of the move to online delivery was that we could continue with the trial rather than pausing until home-visits were permitted. Further still, moving to online delivery meant we could expand our recruitment reach by being able to recruit nationally, rather than just in the cities where our research teams were located. This change in plan enabled us to recruit more quickly in some countries.

FIVE PHASES OF CLINICAL TRIAL PROJECT MANAGEMENT

Clinical trial project management comprises of five main project phases—the initiation of the trial, planning the trial, execution of the trial, monitoring the trial, and closing the trial (Farrell et al., 2010). The *initiating phase* comprises of developing the project idea either solely by the principal investigator or together with a group of researchers. During this period, the research team clarify what is known/unknown about the concept, and liaise with stakeholders and with consumer groups to determine the need for the research. This is important to ensure the research team do not invest considerable time (and money) into research that is not needed and create research waste.

Once the project has been initiated and funding secured, the second phase begins. The *planning phase* can be regarded as one of the most critical in the success of the trial, because if the planning is not comprehensive, potential omissions or risks to the execution of the plan will not be identified, and the project is therefore at risk of failure. As I detail also in Chapter 5, a significant proportion of time should be spent on the planning phase, with a clear set of tasks and timelines outlined to keep the project on track.

In the planning phase of the project, the team identifies how the project will be implemented on a day-to-day basis including who will be responsible for the different activities. The planning phase also includes staff recruitment (and training), establishing communication protocols between the research team (and sub-teams if relevant), plans for recruitment and monitoring recruitment (Chapter 6), data management (Chapter 7), governance structures (Chapter 3), promotion/awareness raising, safety reporting, analysis (Chapter 3), intellectual property and commercialisation (where relevant, Chapter 11), budget management (Chapter 5), and report writing and dissemination (Chapter 10).

Start the planning phase as early as possible. The planning phase for MATCH implementation began 6 months before the funding even commenced (Chapter 1). We established a leadership group which comprised the project manager, the principal investigator, the lead investigators of four different workstreams, and the leader of the capacity building component of the project. We met two-three weekly, planning all aspects of the first phase of the project including formulating a detailed Gantt chart and looking closely at how each of the four workstreams would work together. There were many interdependencies. For example, workstream 2 could not co-design the MATCH app interface without workstream 1 having completed its content design. Workstream 4 could not test the feasibility and acceptability of the wearable sensors until workstream 3 had set up data capture systems where the sensor data would be collected and stored. Further, with such a huge interdisciplinary team comprising creative arts therapists, clinician researchers (psychiatry, physiotherapy, speech pathology, neuropsychology), app designers, software and hardware engineers, health economists, and biostatisticians, establishing understandings of each other's needs, trying to find a common language, and having the broader team understand the music therapy team's vision, were needed early on to ensure that some of the project team's work did not move away from the core aims.

We organised multi-institutional agreements with our partner organisations, organised our intellectual property agreements, developed policies such as the publication policy (Chapter 10), developed risk assessments, organised a press-release to raise awareness of the project, contracted an external party to undertake a branding, logo, and project web design exercise, and consulted with an external party around business development and commercialisation of our MATCH product (Chapter 11). All these components were critical to the success of the project and needed to be planned.

We developed the protocol for the first of 9 studies and submitted an ethics application for these. In planning the first project for MATCH, we needed to flesh out the details of the protocol, select and create assessment tools, develop content for the MATCH app, and have it programmed for initial testing. We engaged a series of consumers to look at the preliminary prototype of the app before field testing it in participants' homes. We applied for ethics, developed Case Report Forms (CRFs), and translated these into electronic CRFs via REDCap (see Chapter 7).

Once the plans have been developed, the project moves into the *execution phase*—essentially, executing the plan. Management involves team members performing their tasks according to the plan. To ensure the plan moves forward, the principal investigator and project manager should meet regularly with the other investigators to provide oversight in to how the trial is tracking and to share details of other aspects of the trial that may be necessary for the investigators to perform their roles and reach their goals. Regular team meetings can help ensure the investigators feel part of the bigger project, ensure they do not work in silos, and ignite enthusiasm for the whole team vision. Similarly, during the execution phase, it can be important to maintain relationships with stakeholders and/or with staff at clinical sites where the project is being implemented. Regular contact and showing appreciation of their involvement will assist in keeping stakeholders and site staff engaged with and committed to the project.

Once the project is underway, we enter the *monitoring and controlling phase* of the project. Here, it will be important to monitor all aspects of the project and adjust the initial plan as needed. Adjustments might be related to the scope, schedule, resource use, communication, or risks associated with the project (ISAC & IFAR, 2018). Several tools which are described later in this chapter and other chapters to assist with monitoring may include creating templates for tracking enrolment, attendance at creative arts therapies sessions, protocol adherence, and maintenance of protocol amendments and procedures. Generating and reviewing data quality reports are also necessary to ensure completeness of the data and protocol adherence. Finally, the *closing phase* of the project involves database lockdown, final decisions on the analysis plan, analysis, and reporting.

Successful Management Approaches

From my perspective, I have found that there are five components to clinical trial management that lead to success. These are managing meetings, team communication and activity, early diagnosis and resolution of problems, creation of efficient systems and processes, accountability, and management of risk.

Good Communication Is Like the Oil in Your Engine

As articulated in Chapter 4, the success of the project is largely dependent upon teamwork and the experience, expertise, and commitment of the research team. However, even when those three boxes are ticked, the project can fail if the team activity is not coordinated. And coordination relies heavily on communication—communication between the principal investigator and project manager and individual researchers, and between researchers. Good communication is like the oil in your engine. It keeps the tractor running so taking care of crops and harvesting can occur efficiently and without a breakdown.

Regular efficient and effective communication will assist members of the research team to feel involved. I cannot stress the words "regular, efficient, and effective" enough. All researchers are busy, they may be involved in other projects with competing interests or may have university teaching and/or administrative and/or clinical commitments to balance as well, so clear and succinct messaging is paramount. Further, listening to and collaboratively helping them to resolve any problems can increase confidence in the principal investigator's capability to lead the trial, and help the research team to feel valued and supported.

My experience thus far is that establishing clear communication strategies at the outset will assist the project team to understand what is needed and expected in project implementation. There are several management approaches that enable clear communication although the success of the approaches taken will depend upon the size and needs of the research team and research project.

Avoid Meeting Madness

As the principal investigator, I spend a significant amount of my time in meetings. In fact, when I review my calendar each week, I find myself involved in approximately three to four research project meetings a day (leadership meetings, meetings with a subset of the full team, with individual researchers, human resources department, finance, research office, external relations, media, ethics, IP/legal, business development, meetings with biostatisticians, etc.). This can make the role of the principal investigator challenging because at times you may find that you spend more time in meetings than actioning any tasks. At times, it is meeting madness. However, while I do experience frustration at meeting-overload, meetings are important not only to efficiently discuss and decide on strategies to resolve or mitigate challenges but also to build strong relationships within the team, promote inclusion and a sense of belonging and ownership of the project, it can be a medium for feedback and continuous improvement.

While regular meetings can be a faster way to discuss important aspects of the trial and can minimise the need for emails, the meetings need to be well coordinated so they are efficient. Setting clear agendas and any pre-reading/meeting preparation distributed ahead of the meeting can facilitate the flow and efficiency of the meetings. It can be helpful for various members of the team to submit progress reports that can be read prior to the meeting and only list agenda items for specific issues that need discussion. Everything else that is "for your information only" can be communicated in a report and does not need meeting time to discuss.

During my leadership of HOMESIDE, the country leaders of the five participating countries met monthly to discuss progress and address issues arising within and across countries. We initially had set agenda items to discuss each month, with a section for new business and business arising from the previous meeting. We had set an initial meeting time of one hour per month to discuss items on the agenda. However, we noted that we often did not get through the agenda items listed, and we felt that many discussions were "rushed" due to the hour-timeframe, thereby leaving us needing to continue the dialogues over email. Inevitably, due to the asynchronous nature of emails, what could have been decided in an additional 10-minute meeting conversation resulted in long email exchanges, sometimes taking up to three weeks to arrive at a decision. This was not an efficient use of our time, and implementing the decisions made was delayed as a result. Therefore, we decided to extend our monthly meetings to 1½ hours, thereby increasing our efficiencies. Further, as we met on zoom, we were better able to "read" each other's responses (facial expression, tone of speech), so we were better able to attune to one another's perspectives. We found email dialogues sometimes led to miscommunication, which is not surprising given cultural differences and when working with people with non-English native speaking languages.

My experiences with the MATCH project were similar. Initially, our fortnightly leadership meetings (meetings with the project leader, project manager, four workstream leaders, and the leader of the capacity building committee) were held every two to three weeks. Like HOMESIDE, we established set agenda items as well as additional issues to discuss as they arose. And like HOMESIDE, we were never able to make our way through the entire agenda. I rectified this quickly by taking on a new approach, one I had not tried before. This was to set agendas with high priority items, low priority items, items that could be held over to subsequent meetings if time did not allow for discussion, and items just for noting/information sharing. This gave the meeting a focus and an opportunity to understand which items required more time for discussion and where decisions needed to be made with reasonable urgency (priority items). We have found the meetings much more efficient because of this reorganisation. However, with all this in mind, I believe that every research team is different, and these are just a few of the models that could be appropriate for a team. Therefore, the principal investigator can take some time to experiment with the structure of meetings to find out which one is best fitting for the project team. It is highly likely that the approach may also change over time. For example, one approach early in the trial might be to have a strong focus on operational issues. As the trial prepares for implementation, there may be multiple items on the agenda where a team decision is needed. Therefore, the meeting is very action focused. However, later in the trial, when in the data collection and monitoring phase, agenda items may be fewer which leaves space and time for more in-depth discussions. This evolution of agenda structures is well illustrated in our HOMESIDE meetings. Two years into the data collection phase of the trial, we moved from operational discussions, such as managing our therapists delivering interventions and on recruitment strategies, to discussing experiences of managing the process of data collection and observations in the demographic data. For example, in September 2021, when we had randomised 60% of our sample, we explored the demographic differences across different countries. We would discuss why Poland, for example, had predominantly adult child carers caring for the person living with dementia (75% of their sample), whereas in the United Kingdom, there were many more spousal carers (81%) taking this responsibility. We discussed the implications of these quite stark differences with respect to its impact on the success of intervention implementation and therapeutic outcomes. As adult children may have other responsibilities (employment, caring for their young children, etc.), they may have less time available to implement the music interventions, and therefore, the impact of the interventions may consequently be smaller in Poland.

Documentation Avoids Miscommunication

Creating relevant documents to guide the trial is also a way to manage communication. The larger and more complex the trial, the greater the need for documents as it can be near impossible to hold all the details of the trial's procedures in human memory. Documents are needed to ensure good recording of data, decisions, policies, and processes.

A good filing system is needed to manage the documents, and where possible, the filing system should be managed by a single person. This is because projects can have several concurrent activities in motion and keeping track of where to locate documents related to different activities can be challenging. As various members of the research team are responsible for different components of the trial, they will undoubtedly be creating documents and needing them to file them in a place accessible for other team members. But how can other members of the team find the documents they wish to access? It is certainly not as straight forward as it may sound because each member of the research team is a unique human being with their own set of logic about where to file and how to name a specific document. As new documents are created, named, and filed by different people, it can become near impossible to find anything quickly and easily. I know several times I have tried to find documents I know exist but because they were not created by myself, they were not found in the folders and subfolders I had expected. Even the search file function may not be helpful if the document is not named in a way that would assist me in finding it.

Let us take the HOMESIDE study as a good example. At the time of writing this chapter, we had a total of 3,173 files and 123 folders with more than 12 months remaining in the trial. Because some researchers needed to be masked from data and some files were confidential and were to be only accessible to a specific subset of the research team, we managed this by establishing four main folders:

- A *general folder* that included subfolders for assessment measures, a data analysis folder, ethics, supervision of therapists, branding and logos, presentations, publications, recruitment, database documents, literature and references, and sub-projects.
- A *management folder* we included folders about budgets, international agreements, grant submission data, committees, patient and public involvement documents, and timelines, milestones, and risks.
- A *researcher training* folder containing subfolders about intervention and assessor training, and
- A folder for the *doctoral program*.

We initially tried to keep a list of every document we created in a document library but as we were adding documents constantly this quickly became unfeasible. After frustrations expressed by several members of the team, we assigned one member of the team to "clean up" our shared folders and organise the documents.

What's Happening Today: Calendar Management

Managing calendars is also an important part of effective trial coordination. When a trial protocol specifies exact timing of participant activities post-randomisation, calendars can be used to schedule participants' intervention sessions, assessment sessions, and interviews. Some database software (e.g. REDCap, Chapter 7) include calendars that can be visible to the relevant team members so the whole team are able to keep a track of participants' flow through the study. For those members of the team who need to remain masked to condition, they can view only calendar entries relevant to them. Colour coding within these calendars can help the project manager and principal investigator identify which team member is performing a task at any one time.

Calendars detailing staff leave can also assist with project planning. Being able to plan staffing for peaks and troughs in specific components of the trial will enable the most efficient use of budget resources. Importantly, a minimum number of staff should always be available to undertake key tasks to avoid lost opportunities (e.g. enrolling participants expressing interest in the study) and crises (assessors are not available to assess during windows stated by the protocol). In my HOMESIDE trial, I initially made an error of not having oversight of when staff involved with the Australian cohort had planned to take leave over the summer vacation. Without realising it until it was too late, we had a gap of about 3 weeks over Christmas and into January where we had insufficient staff coverage. Here's how the series of unexpected events unfolded. (1) Staff had submitted leave applications, not all at the same time, which I approved without thinking to cross check whether anyone else was having leave at that time. (2) We had an unexpected media opportunity to promote the trial which resulted in a flood of expressions of interest to participate in the study. (3) I realised that our two recruitment/screening team were both on vacation leaving the trial vulnerable to losing these potential participants. This critical management process was quickly reviewed and modified to avoid a repeat of this occurrence. From that time forward, all leave was discussed at our Australian team meetings to ensure there was always someone available to undertake randomisation, liaise with the creative arts therapists, and respond to expressions of interest to study participation.

Accountability

Successful project management relies on the research team completing their tasks to a high standard, and according to the planned schedule. Every team member including the principal investigator should be held accountable for their roles, responsibilities, and tasks under each team members' remit. Clear position descriptions can assist the team in understanding what is expected. But this is only part of the picture. The principal investigator and project manager need to balance the ebb and flow of tasks acknowledging there are sometimes pressing timelines and a flurry of activity whereby a map of tasks and timelines is developed with careful coordination of who will do what components of them and by when. Without commitment and accountability of the team and clear expectations of these deadlines, the project implementation will be negatively impacted.

More recently, managing staff roles and responsibilities has been aided by activity planners embedded in applications such as Microsoft Teams or Trello to name just a few of the many available tools. These tools can be useful because action items can be assigned to members of the research team including details of the deadlines. These tools often have action reminders automatically sent to research teams via email or mobile application notifications.

Problem Identification and Resolution

As alluded to, it is rare for a clinical trial to be fully implemented according to plan. The more experience I have as a research leader, the more I have become comfortable with the messiness of trial implementation. Trials are not simple and straight forward even when the trial is well planned, managed, and monitored. They never are. Problems can occur at any stage within the trial and could arise from complex team dynamics, underperforming staff, external factors leading to an unfeasible protocol, an ineffective recruitment strategy, unexpected budget expenses, poor fidelity to intervention or assessment protocols, unmasking, missing data, and lack of support from industry partners/staff at trial sites. None of these challenges are unsolvable, but the key is to identify and resolve them early. This means the principal investigator and project manager need to have regular and good oversight of all components of the trial with clear performance indicators across all areas so that when underperformance is identified, action can be taken.

One example of this was with the MIDDEL clinical trial implemented in residential aged care homes. Our music interventionists (choir directors and music therapists) encountered a range of challenges associated with inconsistent and varying levels of engagement by our industry partners (residential aged care homes). The research team had monthly supervision with the interventionists to review videos of their delivery of interventions to check for intervention fidelity, and to discuss any issues arising at clinical trial sites. On occasions, the interventionists reported events such as care home staff not readying the enrolled study participants for the music sessions and instead, escorting other residents who were not enrolled to the study to the sessions. This was despite the best efforts of our interventionists reminding staff of the need to prioritise study participants over other residents when making decisions about who to provide personal care for first.[3] The regular supervisions with interventionists enabled us to quickly rectify this problem by immediately contacting the care home manager to reiterate the study aims and ensure that care home staff were aware of the need to prioritise the "enrolled" residents' attendance at the scheduled sessions.

Essential Clinical Trial Documents

There are several clinical trial documents that not only aid project management but are required components of ethics applications and clinical trial agreements. These include the study protocol, the clinical trial manual, manual of operational procedures, the statistical analysis plan, and data safety and monitoring plan. The intervention fidelity plan (which is usually embedded within the manual of operational procedures), the statistical analysis plan, and the data safety and monitoring plan will all be discussed in Chapters 3, 8, and 9, respectively.

---

[3] I note the ethical issue here around prioritising study participants over others but as these sessions were only twice per week, other residents could be prioritised for being attended to on other occasions.

Study Protocol

The study protocol is a document that describes the objectives of the project, the study design, methodology, statistical analysis considerations, and the overall organisation of the trial. It is the central document that dictates the conduct and analysis of the trial, and therefore needs to be carefully considered. This protocol is often published in a journal prior to enrolling the first participant, and the protocol details are registered with a clinical trial registry such as the NIH's clinical trial registry (www.clinicaltrials.gov).

The study protocol is important to the trial as it provides the rationale and study design so that the trial leads to an outcome and finding that is rigorous and valid. The protocol is written for four primary reasons: (1) to ensure the feasibility of study design and objectives, (2) to ensure that the study design will collect the information needed to test the hypotheses, (3) to clarify the processes and requirements for all stakeholders involved in the implementation of the study, and (4) to submit to ethical review boards who will assess the protocol with respect to ethical risks balancing with its scientific value (UKTMN, 2018). When wanting to publish in the highest ranked medical journals such as *The Lancet*, *Journal of the American Medical Association*, *The New England Journal of Medicine*, or *The British Medical Journal*, the editors may request to see the protocol prior to publication of the study's findings. Therefore, the protocol must be complete before the enrolment of the first participant. Typically, several members of the study team will add details to the draft, but in the later stages, the principal investigator takes responsibility for the final edits. While it is ill-advised to make too many changes to the protocol after finalising the initial protocol, any amendments must be meticulously documented and dated in a timely manner in the protocol and clinical trials registry. Publishing the protocol paper prior to commencement increases the transparency of the trial processes (UKTMN, 2018). Examples of journals that publish trial protocols include the *Journal of the Society of Clinical Trials, Contemporary Clinical Trials, International Journal of Clinical Trials, Journal of Clinical Trials, British Medical Journal, and Trials*.

When developing the protocol, it can be helpful to be guided by the Standard Protocol Items Recommendations for Interventional Trials (SPIRIT) guidelines (www.spirit-statement.org).

Key components of a study protocol are:

- Background/rationale
- Objectives and purpose
- Study design
- Criteria for inclusion, exclusion, and withdrawal of study subjects
- Treatment /intervention
- Methods and timing for assessing, recording, and analysing data
- Methods for obtaining safety information and safety monitoring
- Statistical methods
- Ethical considerations
- Data management plan
- Funding, and
- Informed consent procedures

When developing the protocol, try to ensure the descriptions are clear, concise, accurate, and thorough (UKTMN, 2018).

Having co-authored several published clinical trial protocols (Baker et al., 2019; Gold et al., 2019; Loi et al., 2022; Tamplin et al., 2021), I have several general tips that can assist researchers in writing up their protocols. First and foremost, use a template. Some sponsors may already have templates with all the headings and subheadings that may be needed in your protocol. If they are not relevant to your trial, you can just delete that heading or use the "not applicable" default.

When drafting the protocol, try to be clear, concise, accurate, and thorough so that every component needed within the trial is detailed. If there are errors or omissions in the document, or the descriptions are unclear and ambiguous, the trial will be subjected to misinterpretation by the researchers (and reviewers of publications of the trials), which can have a dire effect on the trial success (UKTMN, 2018). Keep the terminology consistent. When reviewing others' protocols, it's not helpful when the terms patients, participants, subjects, and residents are used interchangeably. A glossary can be helpful for defining terms and any acronyms used within the protocol. Make sure several members of the research team proof the document to ensure its completeness, clarity, and accuracy.

Finally, make sure there is strict version control and archiving policies (UKTMN, 2018). This will ensure that only the most recent version of the protocol is being used.

Manual of Operational Procedures

The manual of operational procedures (MOPs), sometimes called Standard Operational Procedures, is document that is developed during the planning trial phase and updated throughout the trial. It is akin to a set of instructions that help to manage the implementation of the study and ensure consistency in processes and procedures. They are detailed documents. My project manager for MATCH once said to me, "this manual must be so detailed that it wont matter if we die, someone will be able to carry on based on our documentation without a problem". Indeed, another principal investigator should be able to replicate the study as originally planned if they were to obtain a copy of the MOPs document.

It is important to maintain version control, so all team members are operating from the most up-to-date set of procedures. This document does not just pertain to the activities within the study protocol, but the whole project. This includes policies and processes for recruiting staff, governance, risk assessments, development of case report forms (see later this chapter), database design, managing public and participant involvement, management of adverse events, and document archival procedures. The MOPs will list key people responsible for each task related to the project including what, where, when, and how to undertake tasks and the resources required to achieve it. The project manager normally manages the MOP, and any changes must be documented, dated, and changes communicated to the team. A list of key sections of the protocol includes:

- Introduction
- Staff training plan
- Communications and dissemination plan
- Study flow
- Eligibility and recruitment
- Randomisation
- Masking and unmasking
- Site preparation and monitoring
- Protocol implementation and trial procedural plan
- Procedures for managing trial progress
- Safety assessment and reporting
- Data collection and management
- Site monitoring
- Fidelity checking

- Study definitions
- List of Abbreviation
- Adherence monitoring forms
- Data collection forms/case report forms

Case Report Forms

All case report forms (CRFs) should be developed early in the trial. These are documents that are created and used to capture standardised study data from each participant (CRFs, see also Chapter 7). They detail all the tools used to recruit, screen, track intervention allocation and adherence, and collect outcome measures at all relevant timepoints, for each participant. These CRFs are detailed, including the exact script to be used by the study team when administering the measures to ensure fidelity to the protocol and to decrease assessor differences in assessment procedures. This will ensure the consistency and rigor between members of the research team and increase the reliability of participant responses. When developing these forms, try to avoid the use of free text data as it increases the data entry and management workload and increases the risk of misinterpretation of the data (UKTMN, 2018).

Electronic data capture systems will be described in more detail in Chapter 7, but it is worth noting here that creating electronic versions of CRFs and directly entering the data is a more efficient process than capturing data on paper and then transcribing it. Further, there is less chance for data entry error as it eliminates a whole step in the data collection process.

Clinical Site Management Plan

Many clinical trials in the creative arts therapies are implemented in a clinical setting and sometimes across multiple sites. While stakeholder management is a key component of ensuring success at each site, so too is putting in place processes to safeguard delivery according to the study protocol. As one example, our MIDDEL study involved implementing clinical trial over in 20 residential care units, each with their own physical layout, care culture, and routines. In preparation for implementation, we set up a process that included a pre-trial site visit, meeting with the care home management team, and meeting with the person nominated to be the onsite trial liaison person. We also met with other care home staff to inform them of the trial design and their involvement and to answer any questions about their participation and expectations.

The site visit had a range of functions. Our research team needed to be aware of site-specific protocols for safety of residents, emergency procedures, and how to access participant data that was stored onsite. In addition, we developed a site visit orientation checklist to complete so that we obtained all the necessary information prior to commencing participant screening and recruitment. The simple, but very important checklist included collecting information on available car parking for the research team and sign-in procedures (including any security codes required to unlock wards), the name and contact details of the general manager and the nominated study liaison, assessment and selection of potential rooms to deliver the music interventions and any available resources (e.g. a piano), assessment and selection of a room to conduct baseline and follow-up assessments, decisions about possible days and times suitable for implementation of sessions, WiFi access, and access to toilets, and areas for assessors and music therapists to have a lunch or tea break. The completed checklists were disseminated to all research staff who were assigned to that site and copies sent to the general manager and site liaison person.

Once the implementation had commenced at trial sites, the clinical trial manager and the principal investigator need to be regularly kept abreast of the activities and performance at sites so that any problems arising could be addressed quickly. In the MIDDEL trial, there were many instances where the research team needed to contact either the site liaison person or general manager when there were difficultits accessing data or when residents were continuously not ready for scheduled sessions, thereby impacting their adherence to the intervention protocol. Regular site updates assisted in keeping the site staff engaged and aware of this project which was longitudinal (12 months).

Risk Management Plan

One of the most critical aspects of trial management is to assess and monitor risk. As creative arts therapy researchers, we often consider risk in terms of patient risk of harm. One form of physical or psychological harm may arise during intervention delivery. Another form of harm may occur during assessment and data collection sessions. For example, distress caused by asking participants confronting questions when psychological tests are administered, physical distress when taking salivary samples, or fatigue when asked to perform tasks such as singing or cognitive processing.

However, the World Health Organisation (2005) suggests that in addition to psychological and physical harm, researchers may unknowingly place participants at risk of legal harm, social harm, and economic harm dependent upon the type of research activity. Legal harm may occur when the researcher is obliged to legally disclose information either to protect serious harm to the participant, to another person, or to the community, or because they are required by law to provide information if it is ordered by a court or required by legislation. There may also be a risk of social harm. Examples of harm may be the stigma or discrimination from family or a community as a result to study participation. Economic harm may occur if there are negative economic implications for someone's participation such as a loss of wages to attend study appointments or damage to a participant's employability. A full exploration of these identified risks to participants is beyond the scope of this book and is the subject matter of every ethics application that all researchers must submit prior to study commencement. Researchers are encouraged to consult texts on ethics for further information on physical, psychological, legal, social, and economic harm. An excellent text on ethics relevant to the creative arts therapies is by Cheryl Dileo (2000).

While risk to participants is a key consideration for any research team, risks extend well beyond patient safety and harm issues. Therefore, it is vital that an overall risk assessment and mitigation plan is needed at the outset, often even at the design phase of the trial. But first, here are a few definitions that researchers may wish to use in developing their risk plan. I have drawn on the MIDDEL trial to illustrate this.

- *Risk*—The chance of something happening that will have an impact on achieving the goals of the clinical trial. For MIDDEL, having an underpowered study by not recruiting our target sample size.
- *Risk Assessment*—The process of identifying, analysing, and evaluating risk. For MIDDEL, we assessed the risk of insufficient sample size as a medium risk. We determined this via several mechanisms such as collecting data about the potential pool of participants meeting the criteria, and then evaluating that against the evaluation risk of not translating eligible participants into study enrolments.

- *Risk Management*—The processes and structures the project team put in place to manage risk and risk response. In the MIDDEL trial, we set up spreadsheets to track our communication with next of kin, so that follow-up calls could be made thereby ensuring the greatest likelihood of an expression to participate could lead to a study enrolment.
- *Risk Treatment*—The process of selection and implementation of measures to modify risk. To modify the risk of non-consenting next of kin in MIDDEL, we piloted a set of different phone scripts, experimenting with the order of information presented.
- *Risk Acceptance*—The research team's acknowledgement that there is a risk with the consequences that may result, which is regarded as acceptable.

Developing a Risk Assessment Plan

Many funding bodies require a risk assessment plan be included in grant applications. There are many advantages to early identification of possible risks. The first and perhaps most important advantage is that early identification may result in modifications to the trial design that may mitigate or avoid identified risks which pose a threat to the success of the trial (UKTMN, 2018). For example, an assessment of potential study sites and the number of potential accessible and eligible participants will determine how pragmatic and feasible it will be to recruit the proposed sample size is, and whether study power is achievable based on initial calculations. Similarly, in designing data collection, the ideal scenario may not be feasible. Therefore, there is a risk that the project will fail to meet its objective purely because the risk of an incomplete data set is too high. The researchers need to balance a good scientific decision with what is pragmatic to reduce risk. Conducting feasibility studies or small pilots has the added benefit of testing out the study design and tools which will help to identify what foreseeable risks there are to the project and whether the study design can be adapted to minimise these risks.

During the planning phase of the trial, a more thoroughly fleshed out risk assessment plan should be developed which identifies the risk, estimates the level of risk (low, moderate, or high risk), and a response plan. While the risk assessment is the responsibility of the principal investigator and project manager, risk assessments should have input from all members of the trial team as each brings their unique expertise to the team, and can identify risks and management plans that may be specific to their roles and responsibilities.

In developing a risk response plan, the research team need to consider:

- The methods needed to identify, assess, quantify, respond, monitor, and control the risk.
- Assigning relevant members of the trial team to monitor, analyse, and respond to the risks.
- Developing tools that will mitigate risk.
- Assessing the level of impact problems may have on the schedule, budget, or quality of the clinical trial.
- Developing a communications plan for reporting risks to the team, the sponsor, and the funding body where relevant.

Table 2.1 illustrates an example the risk action plan developed for the recruitment strategy of the MIDDEL project.

Types of Risks in Trials

Fidelity of the intervention. As previously mentioned, the types of risks associated with the trial extend beyond harm to participants. There may be risks associated with the trial design, for example the likelihood of recruiting the target sample. There may also be risks associated with the intervention itself such as ensuring fidelity of the intervention. In a creative arts therapy trial, psychosocial interventions are often at risk of not following the protocolised intervention. Therefore, there is a risk that we are not evaluating the intervention that was planned. I discuss fidelity in more detail in Chapter 8.

Other violations of protocol. Participants' experiences of adverse events, attrition, or non-compliance to the intervention (non-adherence) are also potential risks that could impact the success of the trial. While adverse events, attrition, and poor adherence may be directly associated with harm, it may not always be the case. There is a plethora of reasons why participants may withdraw or not attend the planned intervention sessions. Any participant protocol violations may impact the number of participants eligible for the per protocol analysis. Potential causes of these risks and strategies to minimise these should be thought through and added to the risk management plan.

Table 2.1 Risk action plan for the Australian MIDDEL recruitment strategy

Risk	Recruitment of participants to MIDDEL trial
Summary (recommended response & impact)	To ensure that a minimum of 18 participants per residential aged care site were recruited, screened, and enrolled within four week period. The impact of lower enrolments is moderate as it may lead to the need for adding additional sites and extending the timeline beyond the proposed plan
Proposed Actions	Develop and pilot phone call scripts Liaise with site to obtain list of residents Obtain list of potential residents and screen for inclusion criteria Contact next of kin to explain trial and obtain written consent
Resource Requirements	Access to computer Phone Access to site and database of resident list
Responsibilities	Responsibility of the clinical trial manager to coordinate recruitment actions and check recording of data
Timing	Four-week period from initial site visit
Reporting/Monitoring	Weekly review with principal investigator to track recruitment and examine impact of different recruitment scripts

Protocol violations (major or minor) to the data collection are also a risk that needs to be identified. These include possible violations related to unmasking, missing data, data collected outside the protocol timeline, data loss, and the risk of errors in data collection and/or data entry to the database. Planned actions are needed to minimise these risks.

Staff Capability. Another risk theme relates to the appointment of suitably capable staff to undertake specific research activities. Sometimes projects demand staff with quite a specialised combination of skills which may be hard to find during the hiring process. There may need to be a discussion about the risks associated with hiring applicants who are lacking in one skill set and determining whether this is an acceptable risk. In our MATCH (http://www.musicattunedcare.com/) project, one of our four workstreams was focusing on the co-design of music mobile application.

As the team already recruited a music therapy post-doctoral researcher, the skills required of this second post-doctoral researcher focused more on skills in human computer interaction and working with older people with dementia. Quite a unique set of skills to find from a small pool of eligible applicants. The chief investigators shortlisted the "appointable" applicants and then consulted with the principal investigator when making the final decision. One applicant had strength in human computer interaction while the other had more experience working with vulnerable people as well as having the additional skill set of being a psychologist who had researched the use of music for wellbeing. Both candidates lacked experience in one area. This was identified as a risk to the project's success. We eventually made our decision as to who to appoint, noting it was an "acceptable risk".

Staff Safety. Staff safety is also a factor that needs to be considered in the risk management plan. Certain activities can pose risks to staff safety. For example, staff may be at risk of physical injury when working with participants who are unpredictable and potentially violent towards others in their behaviour. Similarly, if participants' physical instability may potentially lead to harm of a staff member. One example may be in dance/movement therapy whereby the participants may need some physical support while moving in a standing position. If they become unsteady on their feet, there is a risk that the staff member working with them may injure their back or have a fall. The risks are real but may be deemed acceptable risks dependent upon the scenario.

When staff travel to unknown sites, there is also a risk that the site is not safe. Risk assessments and management plans should also be used to protect staff from harm. A good example is in our HOMESIDE (https://www.homesidestudy.eu/) study whereby, prior to adapting the study to an online delivery during the COVID-19 pandemic, assessors and those providing interventions would do so in people's homes within the community. Assessed as a risk, we developed a tailored risk assessment that needed to be completed ahead of the visit (Table 2.2).

Industry Partners. The potential for a breakdown in the relationship with industry partners is also a risk worthy of consideration. Industry partners may contribute cash to the project or in-kind contributions such as allocating their staff time to support the project, provision or access to important equipment (e.g. EEGs, audio-visual technology, art supplies), access to spaces (theatre venues, art studios, etc.), or be the gatekeeper to participant access. The level of reliance on a partnership

Table 2.2 HOMESIDE home visit risk assessment

Occupants	Do others live at your premises (not including caregiver or care recipient) or will visitors likely be there during the visit?
	Is anyone living at or visiting the premises known to be potentially aggressive or violent?
	Do any Apprehended Violence Orders (AVOs) or other orders exist that staff should be aware of?
Hazards	Do you or others living at the premises smoke in the house? Are you willing to abstain during our visit?
	Does any occupant have an infectious disease, e.g. Chicken Pox, Measles, TB?
	Are any weapons kept on the property?
Access	Are we able to access your property easily e.g. keys, clear pathways, easy to open door/gate?
	Is there any difficulty with mobile phone coverage and/or working land line?
	Are there any pets/animals on the premises?

differs between different partners within a single project and between projects, and therefore, the level of risk associated with each partnership is unique. A carefully considered risk management plan to nurture partnerships is needed.

Finance and Resources. Planning for risk management associated with financing the trial is also critical. As projects are often implemented with lean budgets, it does not take much for the project's budget to be depleted prior to completion. Unexpected expenses or unavoidable delays in project commencement can all impact resources. Identifying these risks and putting plans in place to address them will increase the chances of trial completion within budget. For example, if the budget reserved for recruitment is expended well before the recruitment phase has been collected, there is a high risk that the project will fail to reach its enrolment targets. Budget considerations are addressed in detail in Chapter 5.

Regulatory Processes. Finally, there may be risks around regulatory processes including legislation, ethics, and policy. Delays in receiving approvals from these various bodies can place the project at risk of meeting timelines and completing the project within the allocated budget. Within our MATCH project, we were required to enter in additional regulatory processes with respect to the Clinical Trial Registry, the Privacy

Impact Assessment,[4] the Clinical Trial Sponsorship, and the Therapeutic Goods Association (or country-specific equivalent).[5]

COMMON CHALLENGES IN CLINICAL TRIAL EXECUTION

Balancing Complex Workloads

Over the recent years that I have been leading trials, I have noticed that there are several common challenges to trial execution irrespective of trial design. Perhaps the most significant relates to the lack of time chief investigators deovitre to the project. Ideally, project funding would cover the costs of a project manager and project team that implement the study, and that the chief investigators who designed it would focus more on management and monitoring of the trial and its resourcing. However, often there is insufficient funding to fully implement the trial by staff funded to work solely on the trial. Not all grant funding bodies award the full amount the project team requested and need to implement the project. Therefore, the chief investigators are often undertaking more tasks and often working long hours to ensure project completion.

Being able to fully focus on a project is also a challenge researchers may face when they must split and balance their time between several projects and other academic duties. For example, senior researchers may be leading two or three projects while concurrently mentoring early career researchers and doctoral students on their projects. There can be a lot of activity and requests for input from team members on any one day. There are days when I have felt overwhelmed from the constant shifting between one project and another. It becomes difficult to hold the details and decisions in your head (hence the need for good documentation!). This continuous shift between projects and other academic responsibilities

---

[4] A privacy impact assessment (PIA) is a tool for identifying and assessing privacy risks throughout the life of a research project.

[5] Therapeutic Goods Association is part of the Australian Government Department of Health and is responsible for regulating therapeutic goods including medical devices such as our MATCH mobile application. Any product for which therapeutic claims are made must be entered in the Australian Register of Therapeutic Goods (ARTG) before it can be supplied in Australia. Each country has their own equivalent: United States is the Food and Drug Administration (FDA), European Union has the European Medicines Agency (EMA), the United Kingdom's association is the Healthcare products Regulatory Agency (MHRA), and Japan's is the Pharmaceuticals and Medical Devices Agency (PMDA).

can impact my ability to be deeply connected with the trial. This scenario is also the same for other chief investigators in the trial. For example, in MATCH where I had a team of 10 chief investigators and 10 associate investigators, each one of these team members was leading and/or a co-investigator on two or three other projects so was grappling with the same issue of balancing their time across projects. While we as creative arts therapists are passionate about researching creative art therapy projects, it is rare to find a biostatistician or a psychologist or an information scientist that is equally passionate about our projects. This can be a source of frustration at times for the principal investigator.

But even as a project leader, when you are stretched across competing commitments, a lack of time to give the project the full focus it deserves and needs can be frustrating at times.

Budget Constraints

Budgetary constraints pose challenges to research management. It is common for grant funding bodies to award less funding than the research team applied for. Researchers therefore may have to adapt their planned budget expenditure to account for the smaller budget. This scenario may lead to some project activities being under-resourced at the outset. Further, budget issues can be exacerbated when unanticipated problems (those not identified in the risk assessment) occurring during the trial which demand necessary expenditure on items or resources not originally planned for. This means savings need to be found elsewhere, something that can be very challenging to achieve.

An example of this was evident in our HOMESIDE trial. The budget plan was developed pre-COVID-19 pandemic. When the pandemic arrived just 3 months into our recruitment phase, our recruitment slowed substantially, especially in Melbourne where the lockdowns were extensive during 2020.[6] We had a certain budget set aside for recruitment, however, due to the slower than anticipated rate, needed to (a) extend the trial end date to allow for more time to obtain a higher sample size, and (b) had to allocate additional resources for a more active and diverse recruitment strategy (see Chapter 6). Therefore, the budget had to be reviewed to determine where other savings could be made and where

---

[6] Melbourne was known to have had the most days of lockdown during the pandemic (Boaz, 2021).

we could reallocate funding towards our new recruitment strategy. We were fortunate in that a significant proportion of our original budget was set aside to fund our travel to the twice-yearly international consortium meeting. Because travel was banned, we were able to reallocate this money to the recruitment budget line.

Poorly Planned Timelines

Another potential negative impact on project management relates to poor planning of the study timeline. Project plans must often fit into a prespecified project timeline determined by the funding body. But this external requirement can mean the project implementation plan has unrealistic timelines. As I articulated earlier, the planning stage can consume a large proportion of a given timeline and demand resources (time and budget) from the grant. For example, even though I applied and successfully delayed the commencement of HOMESIDE by 5 months, it was still a further 7 months (12 months since being awarded the grant) before we enrolled the first participant. We invested 12 months of our time as investigators, and a further 7 months of the grant period paying research staff to engage in research planning, before being ready to commence study implementation. I learned from this process that the more "planning time" you can have before the grant "clock begins to tick", the better. So now whenever I receive notice that a grant has been awarded, I immediately apply to delay the start date by as along as is allowable (usually no more than 6 months).

Poor Task Prioritisation

Finally, problems occur in trials when individuals or the whole team have difficulty identifying which tasks to prioritise. At times, it seems like all tasks need to be addressed at the same time. It can be helpful to examine the interdependencies between tasks when making decisions as to which tasks require more urgent attention. However, prioritisation is more complex when the project has unrealistic goals and timelines; there have been several moments of insight when I have had to step back and resolve in my own mind that "this goal is not achievable, revise my expectations and move forward". In designing the trial, it is important to really assess what is feasible within the timeframe, and financial and human resources available. Sometimes a project scope must be modified to be realistically achievable.

This scenario played out during the early stages of MATCH. I was working closely with workstreams 3 and 4 when we were designing the environmental and wearable sensors that were to be integrated with the mobile app. I communicated to those two research teams that my vision was that the app would be most useful in regulating agitation when the person with dementia was present in unfamiliar environments such as when in a shopping mall, walking in the street, or at the dentist. After some discussion with the research teams, it was suggested that this was a long-term aim that was perhaps not feasible within the scope and budget of our existing project, and that it "skipped" the important step of seeing how feasible our mobile app with sensor integration was within a controlled environment such as in the person's familiar living room. In other words, more fundamental challenges with the research needed to be worked through, before a more advanced scenario of "being in the wild" could be considered.

Conclusion

Project management is complex, requires time and energy devoted to planning and monitoring, and is the key to the success of a trial. For creative arts therapy researchers, project management is a skill set that most have not had specific training for. Increasing your awareness of and skills in planning a project, especially understanding how the various components outside trial design, impact implementation, will assist researchers to manage trial complexity, and mitigate risk of project failure. It is important to remember that rarely do clinical trials run smoothly and cleanly. But good management may minimise the degree of impact that any trial obstacles present.

References

Baker, F. A., Bloska, J., Stensæth, K., Wosch, T., Bukowska, A., Braat, S., Sousa, T., Tamplin, J., Clark, I. N., Lee, Y.-E. C., Clarke, P., Lautenschlager, N., & Odell-Miller, H. (2019). HOMESIDE: A home-based family caregiver-delivered music intervention for people living with dementia: Protocol of a randomised controlled trial. *British Medical Journal Open*. https://doi.org/10.1136/bmjopen-2019-031332

Baker, F. A., Lee, Y.-E. C., Sousa, T. V., Stretton-Smith, P. A., Tamplin, J., Sveinsdottir, V., Geretsegger, M., Wake, J. D., Assmus, J., & Christian Gold, C. (2022). Clinical effectiveness of Music Interventions for Dementia and Depression in Elderly care (MIDDEL) in the Australian cohort: pragmatic cluster-randomised controlled trial. *The Lancet Healthy Longevity, 3*(3), e153–e165.

Boaz, J. (Producer). (2021). Melbourne passes Buenos Aires' world record for time spent in COVID-19 lockdown. *ABC News Online*. https://www.abc.net.au/news/2021-10-18/adelaide-crows-aflw-deni-varnhagen-refuses-covid-vaccine/100547670

Cullen, H. (n.d.). *Effective project management for clinical trials: A business approach*. Imperial Clinical Research Services. https://www.imperialcrs.com/files/Project_Management_Ebook_Final.pdf. Accessed 19 September 2021.

Dileo, C. (2000). *Ethical thinking in music therapy*. Jeffrey Books.

Farrell, B., Kenyon, S., & Shakur, H. (2010). Managing clinical trials. *Trials, 11*, 78. https://doi.org/10.1186/1745-6215-11-78

Gold, C., Eickholt, J., Assmus, J., Stige, B., Wake, J. D., Baker, F. A., Tamplin, J., Clark, I. Lee, Y.-E., Jacobsen, S. J., Ridder, H. M. O., Kreutz, G., Muthesius, D., Wosch, T., Ceccato, E., Raglio, A., Ruggeri, M., Vink, A., Zuidema, S., Odell-Miller, H., ... Geretsegger, M. (2019). Music Interventions for Dementia and Depression in ELderly care (MIDDEL): Protocol and statistical analysis plan for a multinational cluster-randomised trial. *British Medical Journal Open, 9*(3). https://doi.org/10.1136/bmjopen-2018-023436

ISAC & IFAR. (2018). *A Clinical Trials Toolkit*. The Interventional Studies in Aging Center (ISAC) at the Institute for Aging Research (IFAR). https://ifar-connect.hsl.harvard.edu/isac_book/. Accessed 30 August 2021.

Loi, S. M., Flynn, L., Cadwallader, C., Stretton-Smith, P., Bryant, C., & Baker, F. A. (2022). Music and psychology and social connections program: Protocol for a novel intervention for dyads affected by younger-onset dementia. *Brain Sciences, 12*(4), 503. https://doi.org/10.3390/brainsci12040503

Medical Research Council. (2003). *Clinical trials for tomorrow. An MRC review of randomised controlled trials*. MRC Clinical Trials Series.

Tamplin, J. T., Morris, M. E., Baker, F. A., Sousa, T., Haines, S., Dunn, S., Tull, V., & Vogel, A. P. (2021). ParkinSong Online: Protocol for a telehealth feasibility study of therapeutic group singing for people with Parkinson's disease. *British Medical Journal Open, 2021*(11), e058953. https://doi.org/10.1136/bmjopen-2021-058953

UKTMN. (2018). *Guide to efficient trial management* (6th ed.). UK Trial Managers Network. https://cdn.ymaws.com/www.tmn.ac.uk/resource/resmgr/tmn_guide/uktmng2.web.pdf. Accessed 28 July 2021.

World Health Organisation. (2005). *Handbook of good. Clinical research practice (GCP): Guidance for implementation.* World Health Organisation Library Cataloguing-in-publication data. https://apps.who.int/iris/bitstream/handle/10665/43392/924159392X_eng.pdf?sequence=1&isAllowed=y. Accessed 1 August 2021.

CHAPTER 3

The Art of Good Governance

WHAT IS GOVERNANCE?

Research governance refers to the processes applied by a sponsoring institution[1] to ensure that those involved in implementing the clinical trial are accountable. In this respect, the research must be delivered according to ethical principles, guidelines for responsible research conduct, relevant legislation and regulations, and institutional policy. Research governance also involves managing institutional risk. According to the Australian Commission on Safety and Quality in Health Care (ACSQHC, 2019), research governance includes:

- Ethics approvals and patient safety
- Compliance with local legislation, regulations, and codes of good clinical practice
- Legal issues (contracts, indemnity/insurance)
- Good financial management, risk management, and clinical trial site management

---

[1] A trial sponsor is the institution responsible for the initiation, management, and financing of a trial and carries the medico-legal responsibility associated with its conduct. A sponsor could be a university or a health institution such as a national or statewide health department or a private health institution.

- Managing of research conduct and misconduct, and collaborative research.

The governance frameworks are designed to ensure all those involved in the conduct of trials are accountable for the delivery of safe, well-managed, and high-quality trials that aim to improve clinical care. Those parties involved in the governance processes of clinical trials include the chief investigators, trial project managers and clinical trial managers, clinical trials units, clinicians delivering the trial, ethics review boards, the sponsor, and appointed members of the trial's carefully established governance committees.

While management has an operational focus and involves implementing actions that involve the daily operations of the trial, governance oversees this management, ensuring that there are systems in place to establish policies, frame strategies, manage risk and accountability, and oversee all management processes. Importantly, there are forward-looking (leadership and performance) and retrospective (accountability and conformance) elements of good governance (Australian Commission on Safety and Quality in Health Care, 2019). In addition to overseeing trial implementation, the governing committees may also review major financial decisions of the project to ensure the project is appropriately managed and meets its aims. It reviews and monitors the performance and may challenge management processes and decisions if necessary. The committees are responsible for evaluating progress reports, and reviewing and investigating complaints that arise from the trial management group of the project (see later this chapter). Each country or global region will have their own guidelines and processes for governance and every researcher should become familiar with these ahead of planning a large trial. Examples include the United Kingdom's National Health Service guidelines (https://www.hra.nhs.uk/planning-and-improving-research/) and the OECD Recommendation on the Governance of Clinical Trials (https://www.oecd.org/sti/inno/oecdrecommendationonthegovernanceofclinicaltrials.htm).

The governance of trials is not just the responsibility of the principal investigator and trial sponsor and ethics review board but involves the collective commitment and responsibility of all trial committees and the investigators, clinicians, stakeholders, and patients and consumers who are represented on them.

While the governance structures needed in creative arts therapies clinical trials may differ according to the scope and study design, there are several governing committees and institutional structures that are commonly involved, and therefore, it is useful here to describe their role and responsibilities, and how I have utilised these committees. The governance elements differ dependent upon the stage of the project. During project design, the health institution or universities involved in the grant application will provide an initial assessment; this is then submitted to the granting body who sends out the project for review to expert reviewers. Once the project has granted the funds to implement, the next step is to involve governance structures to obtain project authorisation to commence. Most inexperienced researchers focus on ethical review processes at this time, but for an externally funded project that is complex, the governance elements include financial planning, risk management, legal and administration review, and intellectual property review. If the clinical trial includes participating industry partners (such as a hospital, school, or community organisation), or researchers from another university where project funds are shared, there are other aspects of governance that need to be put in place before the project can commence. During the trial delivery phase, governance focuses on monitoring the trial, handling complaints, and reporting. Finally, governance at project closure will be focused on financial acquittal and project outcome.

Governance at Project Design Stage

The institution (healthcare service or university or research institute) may provide an initial assessment of your project which is often coordinated by a research department within a faculty or centralised within the university, or a specialised department of a hospital or healthcare service for those researchers holding clinician researcher positions within the healthcare sector. This assessment serves several functions. Firstly, it serves to assess the feasibility of the project and ensure it aligns with the institution's mission and strategic plan for research. The institution may provide a peer review of the scientific, ethical, and practical aspects of the proposed project and to confirm that the institution has the infrastructure to support a complex trial. This infrastructure includes facilities, equipment, and staffing. The review also determines whether there are any conflicts of interest present and reviews any risks and proposed risk management strategies.

In my experience, the more and varied people you approach to review your project proposal, the better. Many eyes across a project design inevitably lead to the identification of design weaknesses, unpragmatic or infeasible project components, or risks that the project team were masked to. In my university, we have access to experts from the University of Melbourne's Methods and Implementation Support for Clinical Health and Research Hub which provide expert advice and review on biostatics, health economics, and health informatics. They have assisted me in ensuring my design will be reviewed as feasible and with an appropriate level of risk to the university. Other universities will have access to similar services.

For those researchers whose institutions do not have such infrastructure, you might choose to contract the services of a *clinical trials unit*. These are increasingly more popular, particularly for highly complex or multi-site trials. In essence, clinical trial units comprise of multidisciplinary specialists like the research hub I have access to. These can be easily found throughout the United States and Europe. For example, in the United Kingdom, there are more than 45 registered clinical trial units that can be easily found via the United Kingdom Clinical Trials Unit Network (https://ukcrc-ctu.org.uk). They can provide feedback on the research project to review the study design and study power, recruitment plan, and fidelity and adherence plan. Embedding a health economics analysis is being strongly encouraged, and sometimes mandated by many funding bodies such as the National Institute for Health Research (Gohel & Chetter, 2015), and these clinical trials units can provide assistance to design that component of your trial.

Governance at Project Authorisation Stage

Prior to commencement of the study, a series of reviews by the institution must take place before the study can proceed. First, a financial assessment must take place to ensure a budget sign off by the relevant financial authority. Sometimes the granting body does not provide the funding to totally cover the costs of the project delivery, so negotiation must take place between the research team and institution about short falls within the budget. For example, in our studies funded by the National Health and Medical Research Council, a flat rate to fund the salaries of research staff is stipulated as the maximum amount that can be funded. These fixed rates vary according to the levels of skills and experience required to complete the different tasks. For example, a project manager (see Chapter 4), who coordinates the trial, carries significant responsibility and must be appropriately experienced and renumerated for that role, and therefore, the funding body provides a fixed rate for someone with that level of skill and expertise. Similarly, only a junior staff member of staff is needed for data entry and therefore is renumerated at a lower rate. That said, the fixed rates to fund these different roles are often substantially below the salaries scales paid by institutions, and therefore, there must be negotiations with senior management and the finance team as to how the gaps in salaries between what was funded with the actual staffing costs will be met.

The institution is responsible for working collaboratively with the chief investigators to establish a risk management plan (see Chapter 2 for more information about a risk assessment plan). Here, risks are identified and a strategy to manage that risk is developed including appropriate insurance coverage. Legal requirements cover a review of the roles, responsibilities, and accountabilities of each chief investigator and the organisation. When relevant, there need to be agreements put in place so that the institution becomes a "sponsor" of the clinical trial. Any contractual agreements and/or agreements with collaborating institutions need to be negotiated and agreements signed including the flow of any shared funds, conflicts of interest, defining the roles and responsibilities of each institution and intellectual property. Organising multi-institutional agreements can be a lengthy, complex, and sensitive task. I will use the project of MATCH to highlight this. I initiated discussions with the chief investigators at the University of Melbourne and another organisation in November 2021. We (the University of Melbourne team), had already developed the design of the music therapy informed mobile application and were looking to secure funding to develop it further and test it in the field. We received notification that our grant was successful in June 2021, with an official project start date planned for 1 January 2022. As is usual in Australia, all the funding was transferred from the funding body to my university as the administering (lead) institution of the project. Before we could begin work in June 2022, we needed to put agreements in place. We worked through the legal aspects of establishing a multi-institutional agreement so we could be ready for the project to commence in June. This was a long process with many steps involved. First, we had to determine whether the project was classified as a "clinical trial" even though we were not undertaking a trial where participants were allocated to different conditions. Therefore, the University of Melbourne had to first register as a clinical trial sponsor. To do that, we had to have ethics, which can take two to three months for approval once submitted. The challenging part was, because of the nature of the project (a series of projects whose research designs evolve as the mobile application is developed), there were multiple planned ethics applications, and not all of them regarded as "clinical trials". It took some time for the university to decide that only having the first of the series of projects for ethics was sufficient for the multi-institutional agreement. Needless to say, the process was not finalised until 12 months after initiating the process.

Intellectual property (IP) arrangements are also a critical governance process which needed to be completed prior to project execution. The institutions typically have standard agreement templates for this to ensure the institutions intellectual property is protected. In the development of "goods" (e.g. the mobile application MATCH or an intervention protocol and manual), IP is especially challenging when there are multiple institutions involved and where there is a potential to commercialise the intervention program or application (which we had). While it is the institution's role to negotiate with all parties involved, the chief investigators need to have clarity about "who did what", "when", "how much involvement", and "how it was funded". An historical chart of activities can be helpful. For the MATCH project, this felt like an impossible exercise but was reassured that determining IP can be very complex and that at some point we will come to an agreement between all interested parties. The MATCH project began in 2008 (Phase 1, Fig. 3.1) when I received seed funding to develop and provide preliminary testing of the face-to-face intervention (HOMESIDE). At the time, I developed a series of carer-training interventions which were tested in the homes of people living with dementia, which culminated into a publication of the work (Baker et al., 2012). At the same time, I created scripted scenarios (personas) that were filmed professionally to create a DVD training program; however, this was never released. Phase 2 began in 2018 when I led a successful joint bid to the European Union initiative Joint Programmes for Neurodegenerative Diseases, including universities in the United Kingdom, Norway, Poland, and Germany. Together, the research teams from the 5 countries refined the intervention and then tested it in a randomised controlled trial (Baker, Bloska, et al., 2019). The music therapists who trained carers used my previously developed

Phase 1 HOMESIDE Seed intervention developed and tested*	Phase 2 HOMESIDE RCT Randomised Clinical Trial*	Phase 3 MATCH-PoC Proof of Concept basic functionality home user design/testing*	Phase 4 MATCH Advanced functionality + digital health devices all user design/testing + feasibility study	Phase 5 MATCH Randomised Clinical Trials
2008-2012	2018-2022	2020-2021***	Current-Study	Next Steps

Fig. 3.1 History of the MATCH project

training videos to ensure that therapists were delivering the training interventions in much the same way. We also introduced additional features to the training program. Phase 3 commenced when we received funding from the University of Melbourne to develop the prototype of MATCH, focusing on translating the training into a series of modules suitable for a mobile application and incorporating the knowledge provided by University of Melbourne researchers from the Human Computer Interaction department (Carrasco et al., 2020). Unpacking IP was complex because my IP began in 2008 but was added to by various people along the way.

The final step in the project authorisation stage is for the institution to sign off on all governance activities including ethical approvals.

Governance at Project Implementation Stage and Project Closure

Once all approvals are in place, the project can move to the implementation phase, and then, governance becomes a process focused on monitoring, managing complaints and any research misconduct, and reporting.

It is the principal investigator's responsibility to ensure there is good monitoring of all research participants and compliance with adverse event reporting requirements, management of data and storage, privacy and confidentiality, staff expertise, and appropriate budget expenditure. The ethics committee has responsibility for auditing projects as needed and reviewing annual reports made by the research team. It also has the responsibility of the ethics committee to manage any allegations of research misconduct and complaints made with respect to the implementation of the project. Monitoring participant safety is also part of the remit of the Data Safety Monitoring Board which is described later in this chapter.

The chief investigators are also responsible for measurement of performance against agreed milestones and to initiate change to meet targets as needed. These are discussed in more depth in Chapter 4.

During project closure, the principal investigator undertakes a systematic project closure that includes drafting reports to funding bodies, drafting publications to report the main outcomes, providing descriptions of the findings to participants and stakeholders (if required), and finalising budget expenditure.

Project Governance Committees

Other than the standardised institutional governance structures and procedures such as the ethical review, financial review, risk assessment, and legal and research contracts, it can be helpful to have a suite of project-specific committees and working groups that focus on the project's specific aims and goals. Terms used to describe these different committees and their roles are constantly evolving and differ from country to country. The Medical Research Council (1998) recommends that each trial has at least these three committees: Trial Management Group, Trial Steering Committee, and Data Safety Monitoring Board. In addition, other committees include the patient and public involvement committee, capability committee, statistical analysis plan committee, the dissemination committee, project workstreams, groups working on a study within a trial (SWATs see Chapter 6), and sub-projects.

Trial Management Group

This committee works as part of a tripartite trial oversight structure together with the Trial Steering Committee and Data Safety Monitoring Board (Daykin et al., 2016). The Trial Management Group (TMG, sometimes termed Operations Committee) comprises most frequently of the entire group of chief investigators and key members of the research team such as the project manager to plan, execute, and review the project plan. Therefore, while review and discussion are integral to the committee's focus, the outcomes are always action-oriented. Actions and decisions are formulated so it is clear as to whom, how, when, and with what resources these actions are executed. The level of detail must enable the team to perform their duties in a coordinated way, so specificity is paramount. For example, Dr X will develop the plain language statements for the ethics application, Dr Y will liaise with the ward nurse to obtain a list of potentially eligible participants, and Dr Z will book the meeting room and invite members of the Trial Steering Committee to attend the meeting.

In the MATCH committee, we had 10 chief investigators and 10 associate investigators who were listed on the grant. These members made up the TMG. We met half-yearly to review the whole project. We reviewed our timelines, milestones, and deliverables, and closely examined the context where we were not meeting the project expectations and discussed and strategised solutions to rectify that. We also used the meetings as opportunities to workshop important components of the trial that were likely to effect the whole project's success. This is in direct contrast to subcomponents of the trial that could be reviewed by a subgroup of the project. The TMG also had the opportunity to be updated on governance issues, budget management, ethics, and the other governance committees. Importantly, it also provides space for the team to reflect on progress, celebrate achievements, and maintain a connection with one another. For long-term projects, sustaining relationships is important in maintaining enthusiasm and a sense of commitment to the project. Meeting as a whole group is one mechanism for achieving that.

In our HOMESIDE international study, the set-up was slightly different to MATCH. This is because there were many chief investigators and research support staff to manage across the whole team, 28 in total: 9 in Australia, 4 in Norway, 5 in the United Kingdom, 5 in Germany, and 5 in Poland. Coordinating diaries of so many people can be challenging at the best of times, but to do this across three different time zones, and time zones that moved between summertime and wintertime, was, for pragmatic reasons, not feasible on a regular basis. Therefore, we established a two-tier TGM process. At the first level tier, the five chief investigators leading their country's team, plus myself as principal investigator, met at first fortnightly during the planning phases, and then monthly. This committee was critical for directing the project execution plan in its entirety, but from a "whole project" view. Not only was it practical in terms of coordinating diaries to limit this group to the team of six, but sometimes decisions needed to be made swiftly and efficiently, and this avoided multiple voices from holding up important decisions. Examples of issues brought to this committee included decisions around when to cease recruitment and whether to apply for a project end date extension (and for how long). We examined how each country was tracking according to milestones and recruitment, how we managed country differences in approaches, and how we could support one another to collectively achieve our goals. Every country had their own challenges whether it was staffing, budget, ethics, or specific issues related to implementation, the decisions of which effected the whole project. This remarkable group of researchers was highly committed to completing a successful project and worked collaboratively to problem solve issues as they arose and to support one another during phases of immense pressure.

From here, each country had their own local TMG, led by the principal investigator of each country. Their role was to plan, monitor, and review progress and discuss strategies and actions to support country-specific execution of the project. Only key members of the project team were involved in these meetings which usually included the chief investigator, clinical trial manager(s), the coordinator of intervention facilitators, a consumer representative, and the doctoral student (who attended for research training purposes). Importantly, there were good communication and flow of information between the international TMG and local country TMGs.

Trial Steering Committee

Aim of Trial Steering Committee. The Medical Research Council Guidelines for Good Clinical Practice (1998) states that chief investigators leading clinical trials should establish a Trial Steering Committee (TSC, sometimes referred to as Advisory Committee) of members independent of the trial that "steer" the project towards successful outcomes. Increasingly, funding bodies are becoming risk reluctant and expect to see the plan to establish a TSC with a list of proposed members within the funding application as evidence that the trial will be appropriately governed and so that there are predetermined systems in place to manage problems as they arise. The TSC is one of these mechanisms.

While the TMG is focused on implementation of the project, TSC monitors and supervises the trial, and provides high level advice on all aspects of the trial including policy implications, publicity, and dissemination. Its role is to review the project as a "whole" from start until end and make recommendations to the principal investigator about how to proceed. The TSC typically comprises of members independent of the project which is "critical in avoiding real or perceived conflict of interest or bias". Impartiality serves to protect participants within the trial as well as the principal and chief investigators (Daykin et al., 2016, p. 2). They may also include a stakeholder and/or a consumer. These committees can be large or small dependent upon the scope and design of the project. While chief investigators and members of the research team may be present at meetings, their role is more to provide contextual information as requested by the TSC members rather than to discuss and be involved in any decisions and recommendations that the TSC make. In other words, they are non-voting members. It is important to highlight here that although the TSC does have a governance orientation, it is not part of the "management" structure per se. It should be viewed more as a group of experts who are committed to supporting the research team in navigating challenges from that objective stance (Manula, 2018).

Membership of the Trial Steering Committee. Lane et al. (2020) surveyed 38 clinical trial units, 264 publications of international trials, interviewed 52 trialists, and observed 8 TSC meetings, and arrived at recommendations for the minimum composition of a TSC. They suggested the minimum of 6 independent members in addition to the principal investigator and trial biostatistician (who are both non-voting members). The principal investigator should consult with key members of the research team when deciding on who to invite to be members of the TSC. The composition of experts should be interdisciplinary, academics who are distinguished researchers, and whose approaches and perspectives may differ to yours. These TSC members can help to identify or predict problems and offer suggested solutions looking at the project from a different perspective (Manula, 2018).

Membership could comprise of the following:

- Chair
- Deputy chair
- Expert clinician
- Biostatistician
- Consumer (patient and public involvement)
- Experienced trialist
- Ethics expert
- Expert in health policy
- Stakeholder/industry partner

In our MATCH committee, we included a combination of national and international university academics who had expertise in dementia care from a medical, psychological, and a social perspective. We included clinician-researchers who were embedded within the private and public health systems to offer industry perspectives, and we included a lay person. In addition, the principal investigator and two senior members of the trial team were included as non-voting members.

Recruiting members to the TSC early in the project enables the invited experts time to consider your invitation, and assess whether they have the time, interest, and commitment to participate. Manula (2018) recommends that you provide as much information to the invited experts as possible, pitching to them what the project is about and clearly explaining the expectations of their role should they choose to accept and participate. Offering a comment about what specific expertise they hold that is relevant to the trial helps deepen their understanding of your needs. In my experience, there may be a bit of back-and-forth discussions between the principal investigator and that of the invited TSC members to assist them in deciding whether they have the right expertise to meet the potential needs of the trial. Ultimately, the trial will only benefit from committed members so it can be helpful to make sure that the people invited truly understand the nature of the participation and expectations. Where budget allows, you may be able to offer a financial honorarium for their participation.

Roles of the Trial Steering Committee. Daykin et al. reviewed the TSCs of eight major clinical trials and found that there were two main roles of the Trial Steering Committee—Scientific Quality Assurance and Patient Advocacy. With regard to *scientific quality assurance*, the TSC's role is to help the principal and chief investigators who may be masked by pre-assumptions, to be more objective. By offering different perspectives, the TSC can enable the research team to approach research challenges or interpret the data and results in a different way. In Daykin et al.'s study (2016), one principal investigator quoted "If I don't walk out of these meetings feeling like I've been given a bit of a kicking then they haven't done their job properly, that's what they're there to do ... it's their job to... point out the things that we should be doing better (23, PI, trial 5)" (p. 6). In some cases, the TSC may make the recommendation to terminate a trial if ethically right to do so.

Over the term of the trial, the TSC will review project reports of trial performance and track progress according to the project timelines, and milestones, key performance indicators, and deliverables. As this committee will have a whole project view, they will make recommendations on the vision and direction of the project, the use of the project's budget, recruitment, and project priorities. They can offer guidance on where they perceive the project team should invest effort and energy. After each meeting, the TSC will provide a set of recommendations about how the project should move forward, what needs to happen, and the timelines for doing so. These will be provided to the principal investigator with the expectation of these being discussed at subsequent meetings.

The second major role a TSC has is for *patient advocacy*. This is different from patient safety which is the remit of the Data Safety Monitoring Board (see later this chapter). Patient advocacy and wellbeing refer more to ensuring that the project has the patients' best interests first and foremost, not just those patients in the trial, but for all who will benefit from the outcomes of the trial in the future. The TSC may offer advice or guidance on what aspects of the project may strengthen the usefulness, accessibility, and acceptability of the intervention for the very people who it aims to benefiting. Similarly, the TSC may offer suggestions of how to best utilise and disseminate the findings (progress or final results) so the project's outcomes can serve as an effective mechanism for advocacy, changes in clinical practice, and to influence government policy.

Terms of Reference. To ensure that the TSC operates according to its purpose, it can be helpful to establish terms of reference. Committee members need to understand the expectations of their role on the committee including how frequently the committee will meet and whether these meetings will be face to face or online or a hybrid. The frequency of these meetings is dependent upon the complexity of the project, its scope, the timeline for certain milestones to be attained, and the duration of the project. It would be usual to meet at least annually, but some TSC members meet quarterly or half-yearly. It can be helpful to the TSC and the TMG, if the meetings coincide with times when major milestones or deliverables are scheduled to be met. To get the most out of meetings, it's helpful to have an agenda with previous minutes sent to the committee members at least one week before the meeting, to allow those attending to read any progress report or other documents needed for an efficient discussion, any actions arising from the previous meeting, and a foreshadowing of any major decisions that need to be made at the meeting.

Establishing a TSC Terms of Reference will help guide the chair/s and the committee members in structuring its meetings. The document should include a cover page with the protocol title, protocol number, the protocol version and date this charter is based on, and the study sponsor. It should also include a protocol revision history. The initial pages should also include a table that details all committee member, their role, whether they have voting or non-voting rights, and their signature and date of agreement when they became a member. Headings for the terms of reference would include a section on what the responsibilities are for the TSC such as overseeing the progress towards trial milestones (recruitment, timelines), reviewing adherence and compliance to study protocol and good clinical research practice, reviewing reports on patient safety, and acting on recommendations from the Data Safety Monitoring Board, and reviewing any additional information that might be relevant to the study. A list of responsibilities in the terms of reference might also include providing strategic advice, acting as an arbiter in the case where chief investigators disagree over a strategy or proposed decision, approving discontinuation or extension of recruitment, approving the publication and authorship plans and settling disputes raised by the study team, and reviewing manuscripts and providing final approval for publication where relevant.

Data Safety Monitoring Board

Aim of Data Safety Monitoring Board. The last of the main project-specific committees that are crucial in a clinical trial is the Data Safety Monitoring Board (DSMB). The DSMB is an independent group of experts that contain expertise relevant to the field of study, biostatistics, and trial design. The principal investigator and the trial statistician also participate in the committee but as non-voting members. The committee should have at least three voting members. Compared with the TSC, the DSMB is usually smaller in size and focuses more on the trial implementation rather than the broader remit of the TSC. The DSMB's primary role is to conduct interim monitoring of data that is being collected and review it with respect to participant safety and integrity of the accumulating data. The committee may also assess the validity of the study such as slow rates of accrual, high rates of ineligibility after randomisation, high rates of protocol violations, and unexpectedly high dropout rates. When called for, they may provide written reports to ethical review boards about measures taken to secure participant safety and on any adverse events or protocol deviations that have occurred. Based on the periodic review and evaluation of data, the DMSC may recommend that the project be continued as planned, modified, unmasked, or recommended termination of the trial entirely. They may recommend modifications to the study protocol. In some cases, they may suspend or terminate the study early or recommend removing one of the study arms because the study has achieved its objectives. Finally, they may recommend actions to correct practices if study implementation is unsatisfactory or suspicious.

Terms of Reference. Like the TSC, the DSMB will also have terms of reference that defines the committee's responsibilities and outlines how the DSMB activities and responsibilities relate to other committees within the trial's structure (sponsor, TSC, TMG, ethics and others as relevant). The terms will also document the membership of the committee, standard meeting agenda, and reports required to be submitted to the committee ahead of the meetings. Finally, the terms of reference will include statements about their responsibility for reporting recommendations made during the meetings.

Development of the charter is the responsibility of the DSMB and other key members of the trial including the principal investigator. The regularity of the meetings and the degree of monitoring required by this committee are dependent on the complexity, scope and size of the trial, the level of risk to participants, or the risk of trial failure. Ad hoc meetings can also be scheduled especially if the TMG has urgent concerns such as issues with recruitment, flow of participants through the trial, or unexpected high prevalence of adverse events.

Open and Closed Reports. In preparation for the meetings, the principal investigator and biostatisticians negotiate with the DSMB with respect to the contents for the open and closed reports. The *open report* begins with an overview of the study, study design, and the main aims as well as descriptions of the chosen primary and secondary outcomes. The report goes on to document any protocol amendments and explanations for why amendments were made. The remainder of the report comprises of a series of tables with a narrative that reports recruitment and participant data at the aggregate level.[2] In other words, a report that the research team can review but where they remained masked to data specific to each

---

[2] Aggregate data is that where all the data is pooled and presented as a whole and not by study arm.

study arm. Within the report, an overview of recruitment and participant flow through the different stages of the project is reported. For example, figures that capture fluctuations in recruitment over time, supported by a narrative that may explain such dips or peaks in rate. For example, in HOMESIDE, when COVID-19 first emerged, there was a halt in recruitment. However, recruitment figures also highlighted a sudden increase in recruitment rate as the trial moved to online delivery. Further, the German team placed an advertisement and accompanying article in a pharmacy magazine which resulted in a surge of expressions of interest to participate.

Participant withdrawals and reasons for withdrawal are also important items to be included in the open report. Such data helps the DSMB to identify any trends that might suggest there are issues with the trial that are in need of discussion. Incidences of assessor unmasking are also recorded in the report and any action that was taken to minimise the impact of the unmasking. To illustrate, we had an instance in the Australian HOMESIDE team whereby one assessor was accidentally unmasked prior to the follow-up assessment. To rectify this problem, we assigned a different assessor to complete the follow-up thereby minimising the impact of unmasking. Later in the report, demographic data and data pertaining to the main outcome measure are reported at aggregate level at baseline. Any follow-up data about the primary outcome measure is also presented, again at the aggregate level. Missing data and relevant explanations are also reported here. The final section of the open report concerns the topic of safety. Here, a series of tables report the incidences of adverse events and serious adverse events. This data assists the DSMB to identify any patterns in adverse events that might be the result of study participation and whether any action needs to be taken to reduce future adverse events.

In addition to the open report, a similar *closed report* is prepared by an independent biostatistician who has had access to the unmasked data. Here, data is presented by arm but never shared with any of the chief investigators. This provides the DSMB with a snapshot of how the participants are responding in each arm, they can review the size of the effects to date, and they can review the adverse events according to study arm.

Meeting Structure. Most commonly, the DSMB meeting consists of an open session and a closed session. The open session is held with the whole DSMB committee in addition to the principal investigator, the trial biostatistician/s, and the independent biostatistician who has prepared the closed report. Here, the contents of the open report are first presented by the biostatistician. The DSMB members have an opportunity to ask questions and seek clarifications on any aspect of the trial implementation—recruitment, demographics, adverse events, and missing data. Following the open meeting, a closed session is held which excludes all members of the trial team but includes the independent biostatistician who presents the data in the closed report. Here, the DSMB discusses issues related to the unmasked data.

After the DSMB meeting, the minutes are reviewed by the chair and then sent to the DSMB and research team. The correspondence will include details of the date of the meeting, the data has been reviewed, a statement about the findings, and a summary of the DSMB recommendations. In some cases, the DSMB may make the recommendation to terminate a trial if ethically right to do so.

Fortunately, I have not been in the position to date, where there was a recommendation to terminate a trial. However, HOMESIDE did experience a period of uncertainty early on, where there was a potential for this to occur. This was due to our slow recruitment rate during the early stages of the trial. Our first DSMB meeting to review data to date occurred 6 months post-commencement of the trial. At that stage, recruitment was slow and we had only randomised 18 dyads across three of the five participating countries. Our target sample was 495 and we had approximately 2 years remaining to collect the data. That meant we needed to recruit almost 120 dyads every 6 months compared with the 18 dyads we had recruited in the first 6 months prior. A somewhat scary and seemingly impossible task. At the scheduled meeting, as principal investigator, I provided the committee with reports of the recruitment strategies developed and implemented by each country. The DSMB collaboratively provided feedback on the recruitment strategies and discussed the ethics of whether the trial could continue if it was unlikely to meet statistical power. Recommendations about how to increase the rate of recruitment were offered and we were asked to report back with recruitment numbers three months later. Fortunately (although still slow), our recruitment picked up and we were given the go-ahead to continue.

Project Operational Committees
Whole Team Meetings

In addition to the three formal committees, research teams may establish a series of other committees to progress the work of the trial. The three large trials—MIDDEL, HOMESIDE, and MATCH—had "whole team" meetings from time to time. By whole team, I refer to all chief investigators and associate investigators as well as research staff employed on the project. These could include post-doctoral fellows, doctoral students, research assistants, and other specialised research staff (see Chapter 4). Casual staff such as clinicians employed to deliver interventions were not typically included in what was regarded as "whole team" but from time to time were included, especially during piloting of the intervention.

In our HOMESIDE study, our whole team comprised of the six TMG chief investigators (me as the principal investigator and five other chief investigators who were the lead investigators in each of the five countries), eight other chief investigators, five post-doctoral fellows, and nine other members of the core research team who were assigned specific roles. We also included the participation of the seven doctoral students. We believed this was an excellent opportunity to expose them to the complexities of implementing large trials. We utilised this as a capacity building exercise and embedded mentoring opportunities wherever possible.

After an initial "kick-off meeting" which served the purpose of getting to know one another, laying out processes for working together transnationally, and finalising a few of the remaining aspects of our protocol, our committee then met half-yearly, initially face to face in one of the participating countries (Cambridge 2019, Oslo 2019, Melbourne 2020), but we then transitioned to online during the COVID-19 pandemic. Each of these international meetings was held for three consecutive days with committee members having an opportunity for dialogue across a range of project components. Each meeting began with the principal investigator offering a project update. Here, I would present updates on recruitment, publications, special projects, and any other milestones such as ethics, first randomised participants, and first completed participant. It was an important opportunity to celebrate the progress and strengthen our collective commitment to implementing a world-class randomised controlled trial. Such team-building experiences are described further in Chapter 4.

After the principal investigator's update, each country had an opportunity to present a snapshot of their activities since the last meeting.

We created a culture of sharing both the achievements and challenges. It served as an opportunity for us to identify any common challenges that needed whole team consideration and problem solving. We usually set a theme for the remainder of the meeting. Early on the meetings were focused on pre-implementation phase preparations including finalising the nuances of the intervention design and methods to test fidelity. During the implementation phase, meetings focused on recruitment and unexpected issues that emerged as implementation was underway. Despite careful planning, issues still arose during the trial, especially as COVID-19 implications demanded a rethink of original plans. Later in the trial, we reserved time to review the pooled data by country so we could begin discussing any cultural differences emerging in the profiles of enrolled participants. Towards the end of the trial, we focused our discussions on the dissemination plan including dividing the group into smaller groups to work on different qualitative papers that were drawn from the rich qualitative data embedded in the trial. While these concentrated periods of time as a whole group were instrumental in driving initiatives, it also boosted a sense of *we-ness* and reminded us of our common goal.

Smaller Working Groups and Workstreams

The larger and more complex the project, the greater the need to have smaller "working groups" and workstream teams to collaborate and operationalise the project. Smaller working groups can be a more efficient way to review, problem solve, and plan activities. Efficiencies come from arriving at decisions quickly with fewer but the most relevant people making those decisions. Smaller, targeted working groups also enable members of the team who do not need to be present to be freed up to attend to other project activities. Time is money, so attending only those meetings that are essential can be a resource-efficient way to have the project complete to budget.

The way the smaller working groups or workstream teams are formulated is dependent upon the needs of the project and its design. Figure 3.2 illustrates the different structures of the smaller working groups for HOMESIDE and MATCH.

Within the HOMESIDE team, we had a series of project working groups. Some were established at the outset and were ongoing working groups, and others were established (and concluded) as issues emerged during the project. Figure 3.2 illustrates working groups that were whole

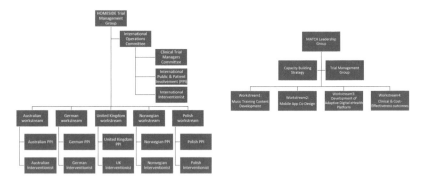

Fig. 3.2 Relationship of working groups to TMG

project-oriented (international) and locally-oriented (nationally based). At the international level, we had the clinical trial managers committee, the interventionists committee, and the patient and public involvement (PPI) committee. The PPI committee will be discussed later in this chapter.

The clinical trial managers across the five countries would meet at least bi-monthly, to discuss issues pertaining to the overall management of the trial process. Issues around assessment delivery, fidelity, and unexpected events were reviewed and discussed. These regular meetings were important to promote quality control and safeguard consistent practices; they aimed to protect drift away from the protocol. One example of an unexpected event that was debated was the concept of "proof of life". One country assessor recounted her experience of collecting data on a dyad (care recipients with dementia and their carers) during phone calls and zoom sessions. She reported that she had never witnessed seeing or hearing the care recipient, despite the carer providing plausible information on their diagnosis. While unlikely, the assessor was concerned about whether the carer was caring for a family member with dementia, with the theory that perhaps the person with dementia was in residential aged care, deeming that dyad ineligible for participation. This scenario was described and discussed at the clinical trial managers meetings as the issue may have been witnessed by other countries as well. They arrived at a decision about how they could go about gaining "proof of life" when an assessor's suspicions were aroused.

The HOMESIDE project also had an international interventionist working group. This was chaired by one of the members of the TMG and was in part a group professional supervision experience. The main focus was on safeguarding the fidelity of the intervention protocols across the five countries so as to strengthen the validity of the trial (Baker, Tamplin, et al., 2019). This was deemed important because each country had slightly different music therapy approaches and were informed by a range of different psychological orientations. While the dominant orientation was humanistic, some countries have stronger psychodynamic and psychoanalytical traditions. Therefore, supervision at an international level provided external monitoring of the practices transnationally, ensuring that the provided interventions were adhering to the intervention protocols. Without this, there was a risk that the interventions delivered would become so dissimilar that research integrity would be weakened. The interventionists met quarterly during the implementation phase of the trial.

The same governance structures at the international level were replicated at the national level. Each country had its own "whole team meetings", as well as a national PPI committee and national interventionist working groups. At the national-level team weekly meeting, the day-to-day implementation of the trial was reviewed and planning for the week/s ahead made. National-level teams included the country leader, clinical trial manager/s, interventionist leader, the doctoral student, and a member of the PPI committee. This structure assisted with the flow of information between international and national-level committees.

MATCH had quite a different set up of working groups because the project was not a randomised controlled trial but a project divided into several smaller studies culminating into a larger feasibility trial during the last two years. The intervention was iteratively developed and then later tested. Governance structures were that it had a TSC and rather than a DSMB (which is typical for controlled trials), it included a Consumer and Carer Safety Committee that reviewed protocols and checked for safety without the need for masking and statistical power. MATCH had a TMG that included all ten chief investigators and ten associate investigators. However, in addition, we established a MATCH leadership group comprising the principal investigator, project manager, four workstream leaders, and the leader of the capacity building strategy (Fig. 3.2). This leadership group initially met to discuss issues such as intellectual property, project branding, contracts, development of milestones timeline, and risk assessment alongside other planning activities. While the TMG met intermittently, the leadership group met regularly as it was the central point for regular reporting, monitoring, discussing, and coordinating the four workstreams of the project.

The MATCH project was developing a sophisticated music therapy informed mobile application involving four separate but interdependent workstreams. One workstream comprised the music therapy team which focused on translating a face-to-face intervention into digital content for home use and in residential aged care. The second workstream led from the discipline human–computer interaction was responsible for designing the interface and assessing its usability in collaboration with the end-users (carers). Workstream 3 comprised software and hardware engineers who created the algorithms, artificial intelligence, and machine learning components of the application, while workstream 4 developed and implemented the clinical and cost-effectiveness evaluation (Fig. 3.2). Coordination of workstream specific tasks occurred through the workstream meetings. However, when major decisions were to be made by a workstream that could potentially impact the activities or timelines of other workstreams or have a significant impact on the project as a whole, the workstream leader brought the proposed action to the leadership group for review and endorsement.

Capacity Building Committee

Many funding bodies expect that large projects and large-scale initiatives such as Centres of Excellence or large clinical trials embed a capacity building strategy into the project plan. Capacity building refers to the mechanisms, supports, and activities that enable the doctoral, post-doctoral, and mid-career researchers to further develop and extend their skills (Cooke et al., 2018). These activities might include mentoring, opportunities for taking leadership roles, providing infrastructure, additional training, facilitating seminar series for them to present at, networking opportunities, and community engagement experiences. It is usual common practice for a senior member of the research team (not necessarily the principal investigator), take on the role of chairing this committee and sometimes co-convening the strategy with an early career researcher (this in and of itself a capacity building activity).

In complex interdisciplinary projects, early and mid-career researchers may have opportunities to "shadow" the work of a chief investigator in a different discipline to better understand how teamwork contributes to achieving a large project's objectives. The strategy might also involve supporting early and mid-career researchers to supervise junior members of the research team and co-supervising doctoral students. It also may include internship programs whereby early career researchers invest time working closely under the supervision of industry partners.

Statistical Analysis Plan Team

The primary function of the statistical analysis plan (SAP) team is to plan and execute the statistical tests needed to answer the research questions and test the hypotheses.[3] These teams usually include biostatisticians and the principal investigator, and other key research team members as needed such as the health economist, data manager, information scientist, and project manager.

The role of the SAP team is evident throughout the trial from the planning stage right through to responding to reviewers' comments when undergoing the peer review process. Initially, the SAP team assist with sample size estimations and power estimations, and have input into the design of the trial and choice of primary and secondary outcome measures. They have a role in checking through the study design to ensure all data needed to test the hypothesis are accounted for. When publishing the study protocol, the SAP team will outline the comparisons and analyses to be undertaken at a very broad level so those reading the protocol are clear as to what is intended in the analysis plan.

As the trial progresses, the SAP team draft reports to the DSMB and are available for consultation around emerging issues with study implementation, recruitment, adverse events, and issues with data collection. Further, the SAP team start to flesh out the analysis procedures, detailing decisions, and rules around how to treat missing data within specific measures. As many creative arts therapies trials draw on many standardised wellbeing measures, reviews of how to use the scores are needed to ensure they are used in the intended ways. Towards the end of the trial, the committee focuses on assessing the completeness of the database and making the final decisions on intention-to-treat and per protocol analyses before the lockdown of the database occurs and no further changes can be made to the plan. Finally, the role of the SAP team is to perform the

---

[3] Details of the statistical analysis plan are outlined in Chapter 9.

analyses and contribute to the write up of the results and main outcome papers.

Public and Patient Involvement Committee

The presence of a public and patient involvement (PPI) committee within clinical research programs is steadily increasing in popularity. Many government and philanthropic funding bodies now mandate PPI committee and the degree and breadth of their involvement are part of the grant assessment criteria in many cases.

PPI refers to a dynamic partnership between patients and/or members of the public and researchers that influence the scope, practice, and focus of a research program (Bate et al., 2016). This occurs when patients, consumers, and stakeholders have direct input into aspects of the trial from the planning through to the dissemination phase. When used strategically and mindfully, the PPI can improve the quality, safety, relevance, feasibility, accessibility, and acceptability of the trial for the participants and stakeholders.

The terminology is ever evolving and partially dependent upon the accepted terminology within each country and by what type of project the PPI is connected to. PPI has been used interchangeably with consumer reference group or end-user engagement group. In our HOMESIDE trial, we used the term PPI as it was an international trial and a more universal term. In the MATCH project however, the term end-user engagement committee was adopted as it was a better fit for a project aim to develop a technology for "end-users" (professional and family carers).

Regardless of whether members are referred to as patients, consumers, users, clients, carers, health and social care professionals, or stakeholders (herein collectively termed "public"), their involvement is distinct to the involvement of people as research participants. Here, involvement refers to their contributions to the project as advisors and/or as co-researchers. Involvement is carried out "with" or "by" members of the public rather than "to", "about", or "for" them (Stanley, 2009). The move towards public involvement in research reflects a larger global trend in movement away from models of government, towards new models of public governance (Madden & Speed, 2017). PPI contributions may be sought at any stage of the project from the initial conception of the project to study design, data collection, and analysis to research dissemination (Evans, 2014).

Frameworks of PPI

As the concept of PPI is a relatively recent phenomenon, there is an emerging discourse around the philosophy and frameworks within which they operate. Early on, Stanley (2009) proposed that engagement can be considered at differing hierarchical levels where participation can operate at the consultative, collaborative, and user-control (manipulation) levels. At the level of consultation, PPI committee members offer advice on specific aspects of the trial requested by the research team. A collaborative level involvement occurs when PPI committee members work closely alongside the research team on issues or challenges. Within these frameworks, the voice and experience of the PPI committee members are regarded as integral to identifying and implementing the most appropriate solution. Finally, at the user-control level of involvement, the PPI committees may work more independently to the research team and provide a summary of recommendations and directives that they would prefer to see embedded in the research program.

Taking a different approach, Ives et al. (2013) proposed that involvement was either pragmatic or ideological. Pragmatic and outcome-oriented involvement focused on providing input into the research processes, outputs, and other components of the research to safeguard the quality and relevance of the research. Conversely, the ideological, rights-based approach focuses less on practical input and more on the "broader social and ethical narratives around democratic representation, transparency, accountability, responsibility and the redressing of power imbalances" (p. 181). In my experience, it does not have to be such a dichotomy, but it is possible that the two frameworks can intersect; both of which may have a more dominant role than the other at different points within the project's time plan. In our HOMESIDE project, at times a very pragmatic approach was adopted, especially at times when the research teams faced barriers. At the pragmatic level, PPI committees at both the local (country) and international levels were involved in reviewing our recruitment strategies, offering their expert advice on advertising materials, and identified and linked us with access to new recruitment sources. We consulted on colour schemes, font, and messaging of advertisements. They provided input on the best government and non-government bodies most likely to result in an expression of interest to participate. And, finally, they contributed small video messages as consumer advocates highlighting the benefit of HOMESIDE that we were able to include in our social media advertising campaigns.

Concurrently, we also had more ideological dialogues about the public's (and researchers') assumptions of carers' experiences and the lives of people living with dementia. These deeper but extremely important discussions enabled our PPI committee members to be more like co-researchers. To illustrate, at one of our HOMESIDE Australian PPI meetings, a carer challenged one of the research team's uses of the word "burden" and articulated that it was a strong assumption that "all" carers experience burden and that there is a need to "fix it". This rights-based advocacy approach was welcomed by the group and enabled deep discussions within the PPI group. It fed into how we framed our interpretations and descriptions of the outcomes.

In a systematic review of PPI in health and social care research, some researchers have raised concerns that PPI contributions are sometimes "tokenistic" and that the PPI exists merely to comply with policy or what is viewed as best practice (Brett et al., 2014). In some studies, there was a failure of the research team to truly utilise the opportunities afforded by the PPI perhaps because they did not have a sound understanding of what the potential value and nature of the contributions could offer the research project. This is not surprising given notion of a PPI committee is still relatively novel, and that opportunities to maximise the public's involvement are still evolving. It takes time to really understand how valuable a PPI committee can be for a project and in what ways they can support a project. Indeed I am still learning how to maximise their participation.

The National Institute for Health Research published a document authored by the INVOLVE (National Institute of Health Research, 2015) group that outlines the values and principles of public involvement in research. I have found their values helpful when considering the purpose and vision of our PPI committees, how to cultivate a culture of consultation and collaboration between researchers and PPI committee members, and to minimise the risk that participation is "tokenistic":

- *Respect* for the public's role and perspectives in research
- *Support* for public to access, involve, and be involved in research
- *Transparency* so the public are clear about the aims and scope of involvement
- *Responsiveness* of researchers in responding to the public's input

- *Fairness of Opportunity* where public is open to involvement without discrimination
- *Accountability* where the researchers are accountable for the public's involvement (and vice versa) (National Institute of Health Research, 2015).

Components of PPI Participation

There are several practical ways that PPI committee members can contribute to the endeavours of the research team. At the planning stage of the trial, the PPI can assist with preparing the research funding application. First, it can be helpful for the PPI to review specific aspects of the application such as the "lay summary" of the proposal. Often researchers have difficulty wording a highly complex study in a way that is accessible to the public. Further, the PPI can review and provide a consumer perspective on to how ethically sound the project design is, and how relevant the project is to meeting consumer needs. In one of our projects "Music and Psychology Social Connections" (MAPS), we drafted a program that involved eight weekly online psychology and music therapy group sessions for carers of people living with early onset dementia (Loi et al., 2022). We were conscious that carers were busy and wanted to minimise their participation burden as much as possible. In designing the program prior to submitting our grant application, we consulted with a carer (who is also a retired researcher) who commented that the burden was low and that carers will value the opportunity to share and connect with others. In other words, we were being "too" considerate of the carers time and that what we considered burden, they would consider an opportunity for dialogue and support. Because of her feedback, we revised our intervention protocol.

Once the project has been funded and the research team are planning for the execution phase, the PPI committee members can contribute to improving the quality and acceptability of the trial, by advising on components such as the use of language and the content of information provided to participants. They can review language to ensure it is appropriate, accessible, non-discriminatory, inclusive, and sensitive as well as assisting in identifying offensive, dismissive, or misleading information (Bee et al., 2018). They can comment on whether the research aims and approaches, expectations of participation, and risks are clearly expressed in the plain language statements so that informed consent is safeguarded. In our HOMESIDE project, our PPI committee members were consulted numerous times locally and internationally on such issues. They even assisted us in drafting scripts for our recruitment videos. Their lay perspective and suggestions for accessible language were instrumental in ensuring that we moved away from academic and clinical language to something more suitable for people with varying levels of education. The PPI would often be the bridge between the researchers and our target participant group.

One aspect of the research process that researchers may not consider involving their PPI committee members is in the analysis of data. In this regard, the PPI committee members can be regarded as co-researchers. This can be approached in several ways. If they are to review raw participant data such as transcripts from interviews or focus groups or open-ended responses to survey questions (all of which have the potential to be identifiable), the PPI committee members would need to register as co-researchers with the ethics review boards, have training in ethics and confidentiality of data, and declare any conflict of interests. They can then offer comments and perspectives which may deepen the researchers' own interpretations of the data. At a less involved level, the PPI committee members may comment on the content of the synthesised (deidentified) findings, offering their consumer perspectives on interpretation and contributing ideas as to framing recommendations for translation into policy and practice. One way I have found helpful with the latter approach is to involve PPI committee members in internal presentations of project progress. In our HOMESIDE project, seven doctoral students were participating in the project and were undertaking various qualitative data analyses. We involved the local and international PPI committee members at all stages during their candidature, offering the PhD students feedback on their emerging project designs and findings at our twice-yearly PhD symposium. The feedback was presented from a lived experience perspective which not only helped deepen the PhD students' interpretations but also helped validate the findings and confirm any proposed generalisability.

Finally, at the dissemination phase of the study, the PPI committee members can contribute ideas about to whom, where, when, and how the findings can be shared to stakeholders, policy-makers, healthcare staff, consumers, and general members of the public. Healthcare professionals and industry partners may provide links or access to opportunities to disseminate findings with those working in the sector who will be responsible for actioning the recommended changes to clinical practice. Consumers and those with lived experience may be invited to review the language describing the findings so that the content is accessible, clear, and jargon free for a lay audience (Bee et al., 2018).

Reasons the Public Get Involved

There is a plethora of reasons why the public may choose to involve themselves in PPI committees spanning personal and social reasons. Many are motivated to participate because they have a strong desire to improve the quality of care for a certain patient group, often because of their positive or negative prior engagement with health or social care services. For other members of the public, they may simply want to have a "voice" that may influence the care opportunities for others (present or future) who are living with the health condition the research project aims to improve. Some members of the public who volunteer for such involvement do so because they want "give something back", or as one person I engaged in said—"paying it forward". By this expression, he inferred that those in the past had helped develop treatments and care models that have helped him, and now he wishes to contribute to better health outcomes for those who may experience similar health challenges in the future.

Establishing and Implementing a PPI

When taking steps to establish a PPI committee, careful consideration should be given to selecting the right members. Try to select people to represent diversity of the sector. By the term diversity, I am not merely considering culture, gender, socioeconomic status, disability, etc., but diversity in lived experiences with respect to the health focus the trial addresses. Generalisability, accessibility, and acceptability of an intervention are more likely to emerge when multiple voices and perspectives are sought during its development and pilot testing. Ideally, the committee should recruit members that are able to commit for a long period, preferably the duration of the trial.[4] Being involved at the outset and keeping membership consistent will enable the building of good working relationships and enable the group to progress the work of PPI

---

[4] I used the term ideal here as in practice, it may be difficult for some people to commit long term dependent upon people's circumstances and whether these change over time.

committee members because they all have a deep understanding of the history of the trial.

The principal investigator should develop and distribute draft terms of reference and member role descriptions ahead of the initial meeting. This can be helpful so that the members can review, consider, and be prepared to ask clarifying questions about the purpose and expectations at the first meeting. They can then make an informed choice about whether to commit to participation. Using layperson's language, the terms of reference should include a brief description of the project, names, and roles of the committee members, who coordinates the committee's activities, who will chair, and how frequently and in what form (in-person or virtual) they will meet. The terms of reference need to clearly articulate what the group will focus on. An annual review of these terms is standard practice.

Some members of the committee may have never participated in this type of committee work prior to volunteering, so will need some training. Preparing a handbook of the project execution plan and timelines using accessible language can be helpful to orient them to the project and what lies ahead. During the training, one of the researchers can explain the project in full, the various stages of the project, and what type of consultation and collaboration may be sought at each stage. As the members may be representatives of the participant group, training may need to be adapted to ensure people with lived experience who may have varying levels of cognitive ability or physical ability are able to process and understand their roles. There are several excellent resources available for researchers to assist them in preparing for PPI (e.g. INVOLVE, 2021; Price et al., 2018; Sheridan et al., 2017) and Bee et al. (2018) have published a very useful handbook about engaging patients and public in research which the reader is encouraged to consult if wanting to delve more deeply into this practice.

Ensuring your PPI committee members continue to be committed to your project, it is important that their contributions are well received by the research team. The most effective way to achieve this is to provide them with feedback on how their input has been acted on it (at least in part) and update them regularly with how their contributions have supported the project, led to improvements, and impacted outcomes. PPI committee members will become easily frustrated, lessen their commitment to the project, and be reluctant to contribute again if consultations lead to no change. At the same time, sometimes their advice and recommendations might not always be possible to implement. For example, when testing hypotheses and safeguarding research integrity within trials, strict protocols must be developed and adhered to and not able to be changed. There is a risk that PPI committee members may make suggestions that are not feasible within the context of the trial plan. Therefore, the research team needs to identify early, which aspects of the trial cannot be adapted or removed, and which aspects they feel can be adapted according to PPI committee recommendations without risking the integrity of the trial. Once this has been decided, it will be important to communicate this to the PPI committee members. Sometimes an explanation for the reasons why some components cannot be changed can be helpful in getting them onboard, so they can clearly understand that the research team have limitations in what they can and cannot change. Ultimately, we want to avoid PPI committee members feeling sidelined, silenced, devalued, and ignored. One experience I encountered during HOMESIDE was that PPI committee members suggest that enrolled participants be allowed to nominate their preferred intervention. A simplified explanation of the concept of bias and generalisability was enough to allay this PPI committee member's concerns. We also assured them that participants were able to receive the music or reading training at the end of the trial, should they have been allocated to their non-preferred intervention group.

On a practical level, Stanley (2009) and Price et al. (2018) recommend that researchers embrace flexibility, including the way meetings are scheduled, located, and their structure and format. It is important to remember that PPI committee members are volunteers, contributing their time and energy while fitting this commitment with competing activities within their own lives and other pre-existing commitments. Therefore, the research team should be prepared to be flexible and accommodate the PPI committee members' needs. This can sometimes mean scheduling meetings after hours or in locations that may be less convenient for the research team, but more convenient for the PPI committee members. I have attended PPI committee meetings on campus, online, and even in a restaurant over lunch. Some are formal and business like in structure, and others are more informal. Both styles have their place and value dependent upon the focus of the meeting, the health status of members, and available resources. In many ways, each PPI committee has their own culture of operating that evolves overtime.

There are many ways of showing your appreciation to PPI committee members over the term of the project. One method could be to offer payment that is commensurate with the nature and demands of the activity. Increasingly, payment should be offered and will be expected by ethics committees and funding bodies. However, the nature of what that payment could be can vary substantially. It may be appropriate to have a discussion with individual members or the group, as to the type and size of remuneration. Monetary payments may not always be possible because of organisational constraints, and if this is the case, payments may take the form of store vouchers for example.

Appreciation of their efforts can also be non-monetary. It is good practice to acknowledge contributions in submitted external reports, posters, presentations, and publications. When appropriate, PPI committee members can be offered opportunities for learning and development, such as inviting them to public presentations on the project, even reserving "V.I.P" places in the audience for them. Holding special events especially for PPI committee members is also a way of highlighting their value. At our half-yearly International HOMESIDE meetings, we always held a session where the PPI committee members had an opportunity to share their experiences, sometimes even presenting about what they were focusing on in their committees. This was usually followed by a social gathering with the whole research team as a way of honouring the PPI committee member contributions.

In my experience of working with PPI committee members, I have been continually surprised by the expertise and breadth of skills they bring to our projects. They often bring questions and concerns that as researchers, we had not considered. We make assumptions about people that they can and do challenge. For example, we initially designed a recruitment poster that had soft images and pastel colours (see Chapter 6) assuming that this was the colour scheme that older people would most likely respond to and prefer. However, the PPI committee commented that they were more drawn to stronger colours and suggested a radical revision of our poster. In essence, they challenged our assumptions about what older people prefer.

Conclusion

Governance is an integral component of every clinical trial. At the very least, every trial should have processes and external parties involved in checking participant safety and for monitoring progress, milestones, and deliverables. Good governance is essential for implementing a rigorous, safe, and effective trial. Governance structures are there to support the trial—a partnership between external independent committees and the research team who are all working collaboratively to achieve the aims of the trial. PPI committee members can bring a new and fresh perspective to the work being undertaken by the research team. There is nothing more rewarding as a researcher, than hearing how the work we are undertaking is perceived by those people who are likely to access and benefit from the interventions once the trials have been completed.

References

Australian Commission on Safety and Quality in Health Care. (2019). *National safety and quality health service standards*. ACSQHC. https://www.safetyandquality.gov.au/topic/national-model-clinical-governance-framework. Accessed 27 September 2021.

Baker, F., Grocke, D., & Pachana, N. (2012). Connecting through music: A study of a spousal carer-directed music intervention designed to prolong fulfilling relationships in couples where one person has dementia. *Australian Journal of Music Therapy, 23,* 4–19.

Baker, F. A., Bloska, J., Stensæth, K., Wosch, T., Bukowska, A., Braat, S., Sousa, T., Tamplin, J., Clark, I. N., Lee, Y.-E. C., Clarke, P., Lautenschlager, N., & Odell-Miller, H. (2019). HOMESIDE: A home-based family caregiver-delivered music intervention for people living with dementia: Protocol of a randomised controlled trial. *British Medical Journal Open.* https://doi.org/10.1136/bmjopen-2019-031332

Baker, F. A., Tamplin, J., Clark, I., Lee, Y.-E. C., Geretsegger, M., & Gold, C. (2019). Treatment fidelity in a music therapy multi-site cluster randomized control trial for people living with dementia: The MIDDEL project. *Journal of Music Therapy.* https://doi.org/10.1093/jmt/thy023

Bate, J., Ranasinghe, N., Ling, R., Preston, J., Nightingale, R., & Denegri, S. (2016). Public and patient involvement in paediatric research. *Archives of Disease in Childhood-Education and Practice Edition, 101*(3), 158–161. https://doi.org/10.1136/archdischild-2015-309500

Bee, P., Brooks, H., Callaghan, P., & Lovell, K. (2018). *A research handbook: For patient and public involvement researchers*. Manchester University Press.

Brett, J., Staniszewska, S., Mockford, C., Herron-Marx, S., Hughes, J., Tysall, C., & Suleman, R. (2014). Mapping the impact of patient and public involvement on health and social care research: A systematic review. *Health Expectations, 17*(5), 637–650. https://doi.org/10.1111/j.1369-7625.2012.00795.x

Carrasco, R., Baker, F. A., Bukowska, A. A., Clark, I. N., Flynn, L. M., McMahon, K., Odell-Miller, H., Stensaeth, K., Tamplin, J., Viera Sousa, T.,

Waycott, J., & Wosch, T. (2020). Empowering caregivers of people living with dementia to use music therapeutically at home design opportunities. *Proceedings of the 32nd Australian Conference on Human Computer Interaction*, 198–209. https://dl.acm.org/doi/10.1145/3441000.3441082

Cooke, J., Gardois, P., & Booth, A. (2018). Uncovering the mechanisms of research capacity development in health and social care: A realist synthesis. *Health Research Policy and Systems, 16*, 93. https://doi.org/10.1186/s12961-018-0363-4

Daykin, A., Selman, L. E., Cramer, H., McCann, S., Shorter, G. W., Sydes, M. R., Gamble, C., Macefield, R., Lane, J. A., & Shaw, A. (2016). What are the roles and valued attributes of a Trial Steering Committee? Ethnographic study of eight clinical trials facing challenges. *Trials, 17*, 307. https://doi.org/10.1186/s13063-016-1425-y

Evans, D. (2014). Patient and public involvement in research in the English NHS: A documentary analysis of the complex interplay of evidence and policy. *Evidence & Policy: A Journal of Research, Debate & Practice, 10*(3), 361–377. https://doi.org/10.1332/174426413X662770

Gohel, M. S., & Chetter, I. (2015). Are clinical trials units essential for a successful trial? (2015). *British Medical Journal, 350*, h2823.

Ives, J., Damery, S., & Redwod, S. (2013). PPI, paradoxes and Plato: Who's sailing the ship? *Journal of Medical Ethics, 39*, 181–185. https://doi.org/10.1136/medethics-2011-100150

Lane, J. A., Gamble, C., Cragg, W. J., Tembo, D., & Sydes, M. R. (2020). A third trial oversight committee: Functions, benefits and issues. *Clinical Trials, 17*(1), 106–112. https://doi.org/10.1177/1740774519881619

Loi, S. M., Flynn, L., Cadwallader, C., Stretton-Smith, P., Bryant, C., & Baker, F. A. (2022). Music and psychology and social connections program: Protocol for a novel intervention for dyads affected by younger-onset dementia. *Brain Sciences, 12*(4), 503. https://doi.org/10.3390/brainsci12040503

Madden, M., & Speed, E. (2017). Beware zombies and unicorns: Toward critical patient and public involvement in health research in a neoliberal context. *Frontiers in Sociology, 2*(7). https://doi.org/10.3389/fsoc.2017.00007

Manula, M. (2018). Why your research project needs a scientific advisory board. *Funding Insight*. Research Professional. https://www.researchprofessional.com/0/rr/funding/insight/2018/11/Why-your-research-project-needs-a-scientific-advisory-board.html. Accessed 7 October 2021.

Medical Research Council. (1998). *Guidelines for good clinical practice in clinical trials*. Medical Research Council. https://www.ukri.org/publications/mrc-guidelines-for-good-clinical-practice-in-clinical-trials-1998-withdrawn/. Accessed 8 October 2021.

National Institute of Health Research. (2014). *Patient and public involvement in health and social care research: A handbook for researchers.* http://www.nihr.ac.uk/funding/how-we-can-help-you/RDS-PPI-Handbook-2014-v8-FINAL.pdf. Accessed 15 October 2021.

National Institute of Health Research. (2015). *Public involvement in research: Values and principles framework.* INVOLVE. https://www.invo.org.uk/wp-content/uploads/2017/08/Values-Principles-framework-Jan2016.pdf. Accessed 13 October 2021.

National Institute of Health Research. (2017). *What is public involvement in research?* INVOLVE. http://www.invo.org.uk/find-out-more/what-is-public-involvement-in-research-2/. Accessed 15 October 2021.

National Institute of Health Research. (2020). *Payment and recognition for public involvement.* INVOLVE. https://www.invo.org.uk/resource-centre/payment-and-recognition-for-public-involvement/. Accessed 15 October 2021.

National Institute of Health Research. (2021). *Briefing notes for researchers: Public Involvement in NHS, public health and social care research.* INVOLVE. https://www.nihr.ac.uk/documents/briefing-notes-for-researchers-public-involvement-in-nhs-health-and-social-care-research/27371?pr=

Price, A., Albarqouni, L., Kirkpatrick, J., Clarke, M., Liew, S. M., Roberts, N., & Burls, A. (2018). Patient and public involvement in the design of clinical trials: An overview of systematic reviews. *Journal of Evaluation in Clinical Practice, 24*(1), 240–253. https://doi.org/10.1111/jep.12580

Sheridan, S., Schrandt, S., Forsythe, L., Hilliard, T. S., & Paez, K. A. (2017). The PCORI engagement rubric: Promising practices for partnering in research. *The Annals of Family Medicine, 15*, 165–170. https://doi.org/10.1370/afm.2042

Stanley, K. (2009). *Exploring impact: Public involvement in NHS, public health and social care research.* INVOLVE. http://www.invo.org.uk/wp-content/uploads/2011/11/Involve_Exploring_Impactfinal28.10.09.pdf

CHAPTER 4

Assembling and Uniting a Team

STAFFING TO YOUR NEEDS

When creative arts therapists begin their journey as a researcher—as a doctoral candidate—they are tasked with leading the whole project as a novice and often as a solo researcher. They will have the support of one or two discipline specific supervisors, and if lucky enough, may have access to a biostatistician to assist with statistics. In some cases, there may be some funding made available to them to employ clinicians to do the clinical work associated with the project and/or employ an assistant to undertake the collection of data so they can remain masked to condition and thereby minimise bias and improve the rigor of the study. However, most typically, without the financial resources to scale up the research, the team is "me, myself, and I". This was certainly my experience. My doctoral supervisor, the late and great Professor Tony Wigram, was a music therapist, and as a scholarship holder, I did have some funding available for some statistical assistance and to employ a clinician to conduct the music therapy sessions, but I had access to nothing else. This is quite a different experience to many doctoral researchers in the health sciences who may be carving out a doctoral project that is nested in a larger study. They have access to an interdisciplinary team which is likely to influence the quality and depth of their research, but also enrich their research training. They would gain a good understanding of the various roles of staff in undertaking a large-scale trial and what research teamwork looks like.

In this chapter, I outline some of the learnings I have encountered from being part of a team and leading a team. It is fair to say at the outset, that without having had any experience of an internship model, shadowing a research leader or benefiting from being a participant in an active research leadership mentoring program, the knowledge gained about establishing and leading a team has emerged from my experiences and through dialogue and observation (from a distance) of other research leaders located in the medical faculty. I am grateful for the inclusive attitude of researchers in the medical faculty who have linked me with potential collaborating researchers.

When planning the research design, writing the funding application, and preparing a research budget, the first question I ask myself is "what are my staffing needs?". And the short answer to that question is, "my staffing needs are to include a team of investigators that cover every skill set necessary to complete the project to the highest level of rigor and excellence as possible". To arrive at this ideal team, I consider the scope of my project, the context within which it is being implemented, the clinical population under investigation, the components of the intervention (including the comparative intervention if there is one), the types of outcomes I am studying, the outcome measures I am including, any specialised equipment being used, and overall management of the project. Let's look at these individually.

When considering who I might need on my team, I first consider the *scope of the project*. Is it a local based study (Melbourne), an Australian wide study, or an international study? My randomised controlled trial of people with acquired neurodisability, was implemented solely in Melbourne (Baker, Tamplin, et al., 2019). Therefore, my team was Melbourne based so we could all contribute intellectually but also practically to implementing the study. The HOMESIDE international trial (Baker, Bloska, et al., 2019), while led out of The University of Melbourne, it assembled research leaders in the other four countries—Poland, Germany, Norway, and the UK. This enabled members in Melbourne to work on the trial implementation but the international team members could discuss the bigger picture issues effecting the trial.

The *context of research implementation* also guides my decisions as to whom might join the research team. If the research is going to be implemented in a hospital context, inviting a researcher in the field who has expertise in implementing research in this context can be helpful. Not only will this person have networks within the hospital that might be useful for the project, but there will be a deeper understanding of how feasible the research is, understanding hospital processes, and anticipating implementation challenges. Other contexts where research might be implemented are aged care homes, schools, community centres, in hospice, in rehabilitation settings, or within people's homes. Each one of these contexts presents feasibility, process, and implementation challenges that can be navigated more successfully when the team includes someone with experience of researching in this context.

Including a relevant *clinical population specialist* can strengthen the team. This expertise can provide a whole gamut of insight into the phenomenon under investigation. For example, if working with children undergoing cancer care, a chosen research specialist could be an oncologist, a psychologist, or a nurse, or if working with people with schizophrenia, the research team might need a psychiatrist. The clinical and research expertise of the chosen team member is dependent upon what is needed on the team. In one study, we trialled implementing a music-assisted relaxation intervention during the transition to non-invasive ventilation (NIV) for people with Motor Neuron Disease (Davies et al., 2016; Tamplin et al., 2017). We needed to include a team member who understood NIV, knowledge about transitioning to NIV without music, how to measure adherence, and the best methods to capture and analyse the research data collected directly by the NIV machine. We invited Professor David Berlowitz to join our team, a physiotherapist who leads research on respiratory support for people with Motor Neuron Disease.

The *intervention* protocol will be primarily designed by the creative arts therapist. However, there may be times when there are components that are introduced from other fields that may call for an expert from another discipline. In our project *The Song Collective*, we are assessing the feasibility and acceptability of an online music-based community program that uses social media, video conferencing and digital music service platforms to create opportunities for group members to share music, stories and experiences, interact and socialise, and develop further knowledge, skills, and confidence in using music and technology as a resource in daily life. As the focus is on social connection, the design of the intervention included expertise from social psychologists. Similarly, in our study *Music and Psychotherapy and Social Connections* (MAPS) (Loi et al., 2022), old age neuropsychiatry, psychology, and music therapy researchers co-designed a group program that combined music therapy with cognitive behavioural therapy (CBT) for people with young onset dementia and their spousal carers. The research team used their discipline specific intervention knowledge and worked to design a program that embedded CBT approaches relevant for this population within the therapeutic songwriting approach (Baker, 2015).

The *outcome* of interest and means to measure outcomes will inform the principal investigator's decisions as to who to appoint to the research team. In our projects, we have had researchers with expertise in measuring walking patterns of cardiac rehabilitation patients (Clark et al., 2016), measuring speech prosody and articulation in Parkinson's patients (Tamplin et al., 2020) or cognitive functioning of people with dementia (Baker et al., 2020), or wearables and sensor instruments that capture accelerometry (steps taken, physical activity intensity, sedentary bouts, body position), vocal patterns, sleep patterns (sleep latency, total sleep time, sleep efficiency), galvanic skin response, photoplethysmography sensors (heart rate monitoring purposes), and indoor tracking as is being used in our MATCH (http://www.musicattunedcare.com/) project. While some research teams might need to include neuroscientists who can employ neuroimaging or EEG techniques to capture changes in neuronal activation, including a specialised researcher on your team that can 1) recommend which measurement tools best capture the changes in the chosen outcome, and 2) where, when, and by whom the measures should be taken, 3) how to implement the measures to ensure research rigor and measurement fidelity, and 4) how to interpret their findings, will all ensure that your study is designed and implemented with the best chance of obtaining complete and reliable data. In addition to recruiting these specialised research experts, the research team will need to include biostatistical expertise, a data manager and information scientist, a project manager or clinical trial manager (depending upon the size of the trial), and perhaps a health economist. These roles will be described later in this chapter.

To illustrate the scope of diverse disciplines included within the research team, I will recount how I arrived at the composition of my team involved in Music Attuned Technology Care via eHealth (MATCH) project. To briefly summarise, we are translating an in-person music therapy carer training program designed to regulate arousal, agitation, and behavioural and psychological symptoms of dementia, into a music-based mobile eHealth platform. We are co-designing the platform with people with living experience, family carers, and residential aged care staff, and it will integrate wearable movement and auditory sensor devices to send continuous behavioural and biomarker data about levels of agitation. Our project will develop a platform that will be used to auto-suggest and synchronously adapt appropriate music to regulate agitation. Towards the end of the four-year study, we will implement a feasibility study in people's homes and in residential aged care, and in regional and metropolitan locations to test its acceptability, usability, and adherence, as well as provide a preliminary evaluation of its cost-effectiveness. We will also test language translations of the eHealth app on a select number of culturally and linguistically diverse populations.

In considering the scope of the project, I needed to consider what would be feasible within a maximum allowable budget request (AUS$2Million) and decided that limiting the data collection sites to Victoria would enable members of the research team to engage directly with participants. Our project context was that the eHealth application would be implemented in people's homes and in residential aged care contexts, so including team members with experience implementing interventions in both contexts were important considerations. When considering the populations involved in the study, I needed to ensure some members of the team had expertise in working with people living with dementia, family caregivers, and residential aged care staff. I included a world leading old age neuropsychiatrist on the team who had expertise in working with all three populations who would be able to provide valuable insights to the responses of our participants, to offer pragmatic perspectives on implementation strategies, and to monitor safety and adverse events. The music therapy training program that was to be embedded in the mobile application, needed to be usable, understandable, and accessible for older people. Therefore, an expert in co-design of digital technologies for older people was needed (human computer interaction) to ensure the design of the mobile application was appropriate for the population using it. Because the core outcome was to regulate agitation, arousal and neuropsychiatric symptoms of people living with dementia, we ascertained that capturing movement and auditory data (speech) would enable us to digitally capture behavioural and biomarker data which would be used to measure continuous changing levels of agitation. This involved including research experts in assessment of changes to movement patterns (physiotherapy, occupational therapy) and speech patterns (speech pathology) as well as a neuropsychologist with expertise in measuring agitation through observation (current gold standard in assessment using the Cohen-Mansfield Agitation Scale). In addition to these clinical research experts, I needed to assemble a team of digital health and artificial intelligence/machine learning experts. I approached a biomedical engineer with expertise in mobile health for people living with dementia, an expert in the use of wearable sensors, a hardware engineer, a software engineer, and an Artificial Intelligence/Machine learning developer who would develop the algorithms to link the movement/auditory detected data with the app and then to develop an algorithm that would enable the app to adapt music to continuously attune to changing agitation levels. As we were wanting to ensure the eHealth application was suitable for people from culturally and linguistically diverse groups, we recruited a healthcare education specialist to assist with adapting the content for other cultural groups. Finally, we needed trialist experts on the team—a biostatistician, a health economist, an information scientist, and a data manager. These roles I will explain later in this chapter.

Principal Investigator

The principal investigator (in some countries referred to as the chief investigator) is the overall lead researcher for a research project. The principal investigator is responsible for the entire research process from conceptualising the project, to submitting the funding proposal, to overseeing implementation, budget, deliverables, reporting, and dissemination. The principal investigator has overall oversight of the project but does not necessarily have input into the day-to-day running of the trial. In my experience, it is important to be quite involved so you can closely monitor what is happening on the ground, where work is not being completed to an adequate standard, but at the same time, to demonstrate to staff your appreciation of their work, showing them your accessible when they need to run things by you, and to assist with problem solving. I am of the view that if you appoint a team that is capable and committed, that a more hands-off approach works best, so long as you are also visible and involved.

The role and responsibilities of a principal investigator vary dependent upon the stage of the research project. The work begins at the proposal phase where the principal investigator leads the preparation of the grant proposal. Usually, the principal investigator writes the proposal to ensure a consistent writing style but may invite other members of the team to input into sections, for example the statistical analysis plan and power calculation. The principal investigator also prepares the project budget and justification.

Once the proposal has been accepted and the project funded, the principal investigator has a range of tasks to complete before the official project starting date. Administrative tasks including deciding who on the team may authorise grant expenditure, organising distribution of funds between departments, universities, and individual investigators and creating a schedule for when those distributions will take place. If working with industry partners or collaborators such as a study site (school, hospital, health organisation), there may be multi-institutional agreements to be signed between parties so the principal investigator must work closely with the legal team to ensure there is a clear understanding of expectations from both parties. At this time, it can be helpful to discuss authorship and intellectual property rights which should be consistent with existing policies and procedures (see Chapter 9) as clarity around expectations early in the collaboration can minimise conflict between investigators further down the track. As ethical approvals can be lengthy processes, it can be helpful to get this process started early and the principal investigator help to drive this process and assign the team members tasks.

At this stage of the planning, the principal investigator can oversee the appointment of research staff including a project manager, post-doctoral researchers, database designers and managers, research assistants, and creative arts therapy clinicians. The principal investigator is responsible for ensuring the team members are suitably qualified and experienced. All members of the team should meet with the principal investigator who should inform them of their obligations and commitments, to ensure that they collect high-quality and accurate data.

Once the project has commenced, the principal investigator's role is to manage the project (in collaboration with the project manager). The principal investigator is responsible for managing the implementation of the scientific and procedural aspects of the project. They will be responsible for seeking approvals from the funding body for any proposed amendments to the team of investigators, use of the budget, project design, or project timeline. All purchases must be approved by the principal investigator who must check that they are allowable, suitable, reasonably priced, and the scientific justification for the purchase is reasonable. The principal investigator ensures the project runs according to the proposed timeline and that the trial is implemented with integrity.

The principal investigator takes responsibility for chairing meetings with the investigators, prepares interim reports for funding bodies and ethics committees (which includes contributions from appropriate members of the team). The principal investigator (in collaboration with the project manager) will draft policies for the project including how data will be accessed and stored.

Project Manager

The key role of the project manager is to be the link between the project's chief investigators who develop the strategy and action plan, with those members of the research team who execute the plan. In essence, they coordinate the trial implementation. Selecting a competent and committed project manager is vital to ensure the project plan is followed and delivered accordingly. The project manager and principal investigator work closely together for the duration of the project. While not essential, it is helpful for the project manager to come from a health discipline so they have insight into the health system and how the project can be embedded into a larger organisation such as a hospital or health service. It is also helpful for the project manager to have good planning skills, time management, and an ability to effectively manage multiple competing priorities.

The main responsibilities of the project manager are:

- plan, develop, and maintain procedures, equipment, and policies
- provide strategic input into the project strategy, management, implementation methodology, quality control, and support for the program
- recruitment, retention, training, appraisal, and supervision of trial team members (together with the principal investigator)
- coordinate the project delivery including implementation of creative arts therapies interventions, data collection, and data analysis
- create reports (in collaboration with the principal investigator) so that it can be easily interpreted and presented to a variety of audiences including the whole team of investigators, the various study committees (see chapter 3), media, participants, and other stakeholders
- interacts with administrative staff of the organisation and external entities to on process and procedural issues

- supports the principal investigator in overseeing the operations of the budget,
- coordinates meetings including agenda preparation, correspondence with team members, and circulation of minutes
- supports the principal investigator in ensuring the research activities comply with government regulations, university policies, and ethics committees
- coordinate the preparation and publication of data, reports and information, ensuring that they meet legislative, contractual, and ethical requirements
- ensure the inclusion of consumer group representatives at the appropriate levels and times
- create and mainten all trial files, including the trial master file, and oversight of site files.

CLINICAL TRIAL MANAGER

The clinical trial manager coordinates the implementation of the actual trial itself. This is in comparison with the project manager who looks at the project, not purely the clinical activities. For smaller trials with smaller budgets, the clinical trial manager may also have the dual role as being the project manager.

The main responsibilities of the project manager are:

- assuring compliance with manual of operational procedures, site specific regulations, ethics, and good clinical practice guidelines
- ensure the timely recruitment of trial participants
- where appropriate, randomisation of participants and processes to protect masking
- efficient and effective data management
- monitoring trial progress to ensure compliance with and adherence to the project plan and to identify, evaluate, and rectify problems
- work with the principal investigator and project manager to ensure that the trial meets its targets, generates quality data, and to predict and plan any changes that warrant to changes in protocol, funding, or time
- create and implement study-specific clinical monitoring tools and documents

- together with the project manager, identify and recruit appropriate clinical study sites
- arrange and oversee site visits
- coordinate and supervise the clinical team.

Some of the skills needed to be a clinical trial manager are an in-depth knowledge and understanding of clinical research processes, ethics and other research regulations, and research methodology. An appreciation of the need to adhere to the study protocol is essential. Sometimes clinicians have difficulty shifting from being a clinician to being a clinician researcher where flexibility to adapt to different participant needs is not always allowable. As soon as processes differ, it introduces bias and may impact the results. The clinical trial manager needs to have a good understanding of this. It is also helpful for the clinical trial manager to have good planning skills, time management, and an ability to effectively manage multiple competing priorities.

Biostatistician

Biostatisticians develop and apply statistical methods to research data generated in health-related fields, including the creative arts therapies. While many researchers have developed skills in statistics as part of their doctoral training or if they had studied psychology at university, the skills that a fully qualified biostatistician brings to the research team is beyond compare, and anyone who has had the good fortune to have one on their team will agree that they can transform your numbers into meaningful data. There is an assumption however that biostatisticians are only needed after the data has been collected. In fact, their input is vital even at the design phase and right the way through the trial as they develop the statistical analysis plan (SAP) (see Chapter 9).

During the initial phases of the study, the biostatistician assists in the design of the trial. They will have input into decisions about primary and secondary endpoints, the comparators or treatment arms of the study, and whether the aim is to show superiority or non-inferiority of the intervention under investigation (Zapf et al., 2020). They will be instrumental in calculating the minimum sample size required to detect effects based on power calculation. They will help to design the masking and randomisation methods (simple, block, stratified, or unequal) to avoid bias, and they will make recommendations on the proposed analyses. The decisions made and proposed trial plan including the statistical analysis should be published in the study protocol and trial registration prior to the enrolment of the first study participant.

During the data collection phase of the study, the biostatisticians are monitoring the data and reporting it to the Data Safety Monitoring Board (Chapter 3) and may perform any planned interim analyses. If the research team plans to make any modifications to the study design, the biostatistician must be involved in the discussions and decisions otherwise the integrity of the study is at risk (Zapf et al., 2020). Throughout the project, the biostatistician is working in collaboration with the principal investigator, to create the detailed SAP. The SAP must be finalised prior to commencing data analysis. In some instances, the biostatistical team will also publish the SAP in a peer reviewed journal prior to database lockdown and unmasking of the data. In the last stages of the project, after the finalisation of the data analysis according to the SAP, the biostatistician contributes to reporting the results and is responsible for the appropriate presentation and the correct interpretation of the results.

HEALTH ECONOMIST

In a world where creative arts therapists are competing with other health disciplines for the provision of services within ever shrinking health budgets, being able to demonstrate the cost-effectiveness, cost-benefit, and health economics outcomes may be the most powerful and policy-changing metrics your study can generate. Health economists apply economic theories to evaluate the maximum health gained for the resources spent (Flight et al., 2020). Economic evaluations are frequently conducted alongside clinical trials (Thorn et al., 2021) and if your funding budget allowed it, I would recommend trying to embed a cost-effectiveness analysis into your project and draw on the specialist expertise of a health economist to do so. Like the biostatistician, the health economist is needed during the planning phase of the trial to ensure the right data collection plan will generate the data needed to conduct the health economic analysis. They are responsible for mapping out the data needed to be collected from participants, from organisations, and from the interventionists, about costs in delivering the intervention, the change in costs of care more generally, and changes in quality of adjusted life years. This data will be compared with the economic costs associated with standard care and/or a comparative intervention.

Information Scientist

When I first started out as a researcher, the whole concept of an information scientist was foreign to me. I was used to storing information on word documents and excel spreadsheets that were often ungainly to work with and extracting data was near impossible to do quickly and easily. But nevertheless, when you are recruiting 20 to 30 participants, using excel is not totally impossible. As soon as your number of participants increases, there is a real need to have a more efficient data management process that will enable you to collect, classify, manipulate, store, restore, move, disseminate, and protect data quickly and easily. This is where the information scientist comes into play. Their role is to do exactly that, set up systems (and modify along the way if required), to meet the needs of each individual trial. To recruit an excellent information scientist, good knowledge of creating databases is essential, as well as good skills in representing the data using graphics and graphs. I always say to my research team, that the only data we want is good data. If it is not good data, you might as well have missing data (and some would say missing data is even preferred to inaccurate or errors in data). An information scientist can help ensure the research team collect good data as the system will be set up to ensure questions are answered in a way that minimises error and that data is collected and stored in a consistent manner across all members of the team. The information scientist will have an important role at the beginning of the trial in helping to set up the database which needs to be developed and tested prior to commencement of the trial. Their level of activity then drops as the trial is up and running but may be called upon to resolve issues, add new users, and train new members of the team in use of the tools and other data extraction and retrieval requests as needed.

The main responsibilities of an information scientist in a clinical trial are:

- to build a database that stores all the necessary data needed to answer the aims of the project
- to classify the data gathered and design reporting tools
- to manage the database and draft guidelines for the research team to complete it, verify it, and lock data collection

- to manage who has access to the data, and what parts of the full data set they have access too
- checks all participant records are filed and provides reports for missing data.

More details about the actual database construction is detailed in Chapter 7.

DATA MANAGER

The data manager works with information scientist (for smaller studies this may even be the same person undertaking both roles) to ensure the data is complete. The data manager monitors incoming data from study sites, validates it, tracks the data, and checks for accuracy and quality. For example, the data manager will review entries to check that values entered are valid, and that any anomalies are immediately chased up with the data entry person for cross checking. The data manager works with the project manager and principal investigator in providing data monitoring and reporting. They can generate intermittent reports such as number of complete entries (participant entries), the number of randomisations, the number of participants with complete baseline data, the number allocated to each arm of the study, and recruitment tracking data including by whom and where participants have been recruited.

OTHER TEAM MEMBERS

The research team may comprise of other members of the team who are not chief investigators but are nevertheless needed to implement the trial. These people may include a specialist team of recruiters who promote the trial and proactively communicate with, screen, and enrol participants in the study. You may have specialised clinical assessors such as a neuropsychologist who is trained to collect the data you need to test the effectiveness of the proposed intervention. Importantly, having excellent clinicians to deliver the creative arts therapy intervention under investigation is also an important consideration. When preparing the budgets, people often say to me, "can't you use music therapy students to deliver the music therapy interventions, they are much cheaper [free]?" My answer is always a very firm—no. In my opinion, if you want to demonstrate that a creative arts therapy method positively influences the participants health outcomes, you want to give your project the best chance of success by hiring the very best clinicians to deliver it. It's not like taking a drug where everyone gets the same. Psychosocial interventions including creative arts therapies should have core components (see Chapter 8 on fidelity), but there are lots of variables that make delivering an intervention in a consistent way more challenging. In many ways, despite having an excellent designed therapy intervention protocol, the therapy intervention is only as good as the therapist who delivers it. So always choose the best clinicians and be prepared to pay for that privilege.

Optimising Performance: A *We-ness* Culture

Once the principal investigator has formed the research team, the group embark on a long and sometimes challenging journey together as they work towards achieving their shared long-term goal. As research teams typically work from the conceptual stage through to the final reporting of outcomes, the team can be working together for three to five years, sometimes longer depending upon the project. Cultivating and sustaining a well-functioning team is one of the most important roles of the principal investigator has over the life of the project. Ideally, the team needs to experience as sense of "we-ness" not "me-ness" (Makris et al., 2018), which can be tough when some members of the team may be involved in multiple projects so time invested in your project may compete with their other commitments. Nevertheless, a "we-ness" culture is possible so long as team members have a good understanding of their various roles and responsibilities.

To arrive at a culture of we-ness, it can be useful to have a sense of what a high-performing cohesive research team looks like, and essentially it is not really any different from any well-performing teams in other contexts. According to Cook (2009), a well-performing team is one that has members who demonstrate drive and ambition, that complete tasks, develop new ideas, transform these ideas into actions and solutions, think strategically and make objective decisions, and in general can see problems from other group members' perspective (p. 38). Bourgault and Goforth (2021) argues that the most successful leaders are the ones who invest equal amounts of time focused on team relationships as on task-oriented activities.

Empowering the Team

Polanco et al. (2011) proposes that high-performance research teams have a sense of team empowerment that enables the group to engage in participatory decision-making. They suggest that empowered teams are more productive and pro-active and that the research leader can get the best out of their team when they delegate responsibility to team members so they can gain a sense of personal control and derive meaning from their contributions. To arrive at participatory decision-making, the principal investigator must trust in this process and have confidence that the research team have all the necessary skills and competencies to do so. Actioning that trust is of course much more difficult than it might first appear, and I know I fluctuate between micro- and micromanaging.[1] Finding the right balance depends upon the confidence the principal investigator (and project manager) has with the team. The level of trust and confidence can vary between level and type of expertise and the different tasks involved in the project. Some tasks will require more oversight than others. After all, the success of the trial is essentially the principal investigator's responsibility.

Returning to the study of MATCH, the scope of the project and the size and diversity of the research team meant that it was impossible for me to have close oversight on all the components of the project. It was for that very reason we established the four workstreams, each with their own leaders. For three of these workstreams (1) mobile app co-design, (2) development of the adaptive digital health platform, and (3) clinical and cost-effectiveness, it was relatively easy for me to "let go" of the need to monitor closely how they were progressing and empower those workstream leaders to go about their workplans. The same could not be said for the workstream focused on developing music therapy training content. As this was my discipline, and as the project was part of my long-term vision, I had very clear ideas in my mind about what I thought the mobile

---

[1] Micromanagers are those that are excessive in their observation and control of team members' actions. They need to scrutinise even the minutest of tasks. Macro-managers are those who have a more hands-off approach and let the team go about their tasks with minimal direct supervision.

application should be. During the development of the minimal viable product (MVP), I was the main driver of its development, seeking input from other members of the music therapy team for comment. However, once this MVP was almost ready to test in the field, I made a conscious decision to step back and let the workstream 1 leader take over leadership of this workstream. To assist myself and her (Dr Jeanette Tamplin) in this transition, I decided to stop attending the workstream's weekly meetings and essentially wait for them to invite me to meetings if and when they wanted my input. I wanted to give the Jeanette and her team the possibility to put their "stamp" on the project, thereby fostering a sense of ownership.

Safety Within the Group

A we-ness culture also demands that the work environment and processes to address issues are transparent and safe for all team members (Bourgault & Goforth, 2021). Safety is promoted through honesty, trust, openness, self-disclosure, and an acceptance that mistakes are a part of how the group learns to work together (Makis et al., 2018). Wherever possible, raising and solving issues should be addressed at a team level rather than directed at specific individuals. When the research leader can foster this culture, members of the group will feel safer to raise issues and suggest solutions.

I reflect on one example I experienced when working with the Australian HOMESIDE team. When first implementing the trial, we identified some issues around scheduling its various components. First, assessors needed to screen and then complete baseline assessments for participants. Following this, assessors notified the country leader that the participants were ready for randomisation. The country leader's task was then to randomise the participants and notify the team member who was coordinating the allocation of therapists to work with participants. This clinical component of the trial needed to commence within 14 days of randomisation. We encountered a problem early in the trial when at one point, we were ready to allocate a therapist to implement the clinical component and discovered that none of the interventionists were available within the 14-day window. They were either already at full capacity or had planned vacation. Team stress escalated as they realised the extent of the potential protocol violations. As a team, we determined that these violations were avoidable if there was a greater awareness of the external factors that might impact the stipulated timeline. Once this issue arose in the team, we discussed a strategy together which involved better communication between team members to ensure that both the participants and interventionists were available to commence the intervention within 14 days from randomisation.

Maximising the team's strengths. When leading a newly formed group, it can be helpful for the principal investigator to take time to sit and reflect on each team member's strengths and limitations, and the strength and limitations of the entire team collectively (is the whole greater than the sum of its parts?). Further, I recommend revisiting these opportunities for reflection at various moments throughout the trial as people and your team grow and develop. As part of this reflection, it can be helpful to consider the types of personalities of the members of the team as these can guide the principal investigator in determining which roles are best assigned to which team members. Belbin (2010), a pioneer in assessing how individuals behave in a team environment, classified team members into three broad categories (action-oriented, people-oriented, and thinking-oriented).

Belbin (2010) proposed that *action-oriented* members of the team are focused on achieving the task. Some are *drivers* responsible for driving the team forward are future focused and can face and overcome barriers that they encounter. Other action-oriented members can be a *handy-person*[2] who turn plans into actions, are reliable, are focused on completing the task efficiently, and continue to act until the task is complete. Essential to any research team is what Belbin classifies as *the proof-reader*. They are conscientious, focused on detail, but are however reluctant to delegate or change. Within the research context, action-oriented members keep a project on track, they can identify when tasks are not progressing and will strive to rectify the issue.

An example of action-oriented members rectifying an issue occurred in our HOMESIDE project (Baker, Bloska, et al., 2019). Not long after the project began data collection, the COVID-19 pandemic emerged as a challenge. At that time, our project was designed to be an in-person music and reading intervention trial. Lockdowns staggered at different times across our 5 countries, meant one of two things—to pause our trial and wait for the pandemic to end, or to adapt our trial to accommodate

---

[2] Termed by Belbin as the handman, I have renamed handy-person.

the changed context. At the time, it was unclear how long this pandemic would continue for, and our biostatisticians strongly encouraged us to "pause"; claiming that if we believed the intervention was likely to be more effective delivered in-person (which is what we powered the study for), then we should pause and wait. Nonetheless, we decided to adapt the intervention and "go online". Four of the action-oriented members of the team enthusiastically drove the actioning of this decision and immediately began to review the assessment and intervention procedures detailed in our handbook. One member who was more of a *driver* identified the enablers and barriers to online delivery, advising the entire team of investigators on options. Another two other action-oriented members of the sub-team[3] were classified as a *handy-person*. They began to adapt our tools, policies, and processes to enable the online delivery—one focused on screening, enrolment, and assessment, the other on translating the intervention to online delivery. Concurrently, the fourth member of that sub-team, the *proof-reader*, meticulously went through every document to cross check everything that needed to be changed in the handbook, ans was charged with revising the client report forms and database. This was a sub-team of individuals who collaboratively worked together to transform our trial to one that was responsive to the conditions posed upon us by the pandemic.

In contrast, *people-oriented* members of the team are more focused on the relationships than the task themselves. The first subtype is that of the *chairperson*. These people are often talented at facilitating discussion, enabling all views to be heard but are however sometimes lacking in strong opinions and rely on others to make decisions. Other members of the team are *accommodators*. They are more cooperative and sensitive to team members' individual needs, are good listeners, and respectful of others. They can create a cohesive atmosphere but can be uncomfortable when unexpectedly asked to make a decision. Finally, Belbin classified *the networker* as someone who is outgoing, communicative, enthusiastic, and great at networking and meeting other people.

In our HOMESIDE team, there are three or four of the team members who would be regarded as people-oriented. Some provided local or international professional supervision of the therapists (the *chairperson*) that were implementing the music and reading interventions. They fostered

---

[3] Sub-team is a term designated to describe a subset of the entire research team.

discussion with the group. These team members were ideally suited to facilitate these groups as they created the safe space for group members to discuss their experiences of delivering the intervention and no decisions were really required in these meetings.

Within out HOMESIDE leadership team, two members of the group were particularly effective *accommodators*. At times, discussions could be challenging with different country leaders advocating for a different approach to the same challenge. There were moments of discomfort. The accommodators in the group were always quick to identify these situations and would step in to diffuse the situation, enabling the group to reflect on their views in the moment and approach a decision more collaboratively.

Lastly, we had several *networkers* within our team. They worked with our patient and public involvement group (Chapter 3), industry partners, and planned social events at our international meetings that brought the team together to share fun, music, and cultural experiences, and debrief. This offered the whole team an opportunity to relax and get to know each other on a more personal level. When working internationally, this was helpful in enabling us all to establish a deep respect and appreciation of one another and the nuanced contexts of each country's participation.

Belbin's (2010) final category of team members are those that are *thinking* team members. The first is the *evaluator*, a strategic thinker who has strengths in examining all the options while being realistic and astute. This team member has limitation in that at times appears to be uninspiring, cautious, and slow to change. This is contrast to Belin's final personality, the *ideas person*. This person is creative and often unorthodox, allowing the team to consider perspectives that may be outside the research paradigm. Often the ideas are initially perceived as unrealistic and impractical, however, can "open" the team to consider previously taboo options. Within our HOMESIDE leadership team, we had an *evaluator* and an *ideas person*. When both were engaged in problem solving, the decision and subsequent actions always solved the issue.

In essence, having a team with a mix of all these personalities leads to an agile team that is responsive to the numerous challenges that will undoubtedly occur at various stages throughout the clinical trial. If you are already a principal investigator or a member of any research team, you can probably identify people who fit (although perhaps not neatly) into these categories. Within a research team context, it is important to foster the strengths of each while maintaining cohesion. I have witnessed team members becoming frustrated with one other when clashes of ideas and approaches to the project are brought to the fore. A good principal investigator is instrumental in assisting the team to navigate these conflicts and helping them learn to appreciate their diversity in strengths.

Leading the Team

The role of the principal investigator goes beyond just fostering good relationships. The principal investigator needs to lead the team, challenging them while balancing this with providing advice, guidance, and positive feedback. Challenge may entail encouraging the team members to reflect on their actions and decisions using probing questions, to offer alternative ideas, or to set goals that "stretch" them but highlight the positive benefits of meeting those goals. Recruitment was the biggest barrier to the success of the HOMESIDE trial. As the principal investigator, I noted early on that recruitment was falling behind schedule and that the task of meeting our target sample size within the available timeframe was becoming increasingly more challenging. I decided to implement strategies to challenge the 5 country teams. One of them was that they had to generate a fortnightly report that indicated how many people had expressed interest in participating, how many had signed up, and how many were randomised. Each country was expected to reach a minimum of 5 per month. In addition to this, their fortnightly report had to detail what recruitment activities their team had engaged in whether that was emailing organisations, approaching people through databases, (online) presentations, etc. (see Chapter 6). The anticipation of that regular reporting activated the teams to consistently meet and discuss recruitment options and act on them. But this was not a one-way reporting exercise. I made a concerted effort to celebrate what might be viewed as even the smallest of achievements. When different countries exceeded a monthly target, I would congratulate to the whole team. Similarly, as milestones were met—first 10 dyads, 25 dyads, 50 dyads, and whole sample, I would send congratulatory emails and acknowledge in meetings their efforts. These small acts of encouragement are important in maintaining their stamina to continue thire efforts towards achieving the sample target.

Conclusion

Having the right team to meet your needs is a fundamental need to ensuring your project is well designed, implemented, and reported. It is the principal investigator's role to ensure that all expertise is covered within the assembled team. However, this alone does not lead to success. Considered leadership which creates a cohesive team and allows members to utilise their strengths will ensure the team works as a united group towards their common goal. When people ask me about what I enjoy most about my research endeavours, I always respond with "leading a great team". There is nothing more rewarding than assembling, leading, and supporting an enthusiastic, committed, talented, and diverse team that is confident, capable, and agile to respond to the very many barriers encountered along the way.

References

Baker, F. A. (2015). *Therapeutic songwriting: Developments in theory, methods, and practice.* Palgrave Macmillan.

Baker, F. A., Bloska, J., Stensæth, K., Wosch, T., Bukowska, A., Braat, S., Sousa, T., Tamplin, J., Clark, I. N., Lee, Y.-E. C., Clarke, P., Lautenschlager, N., & Odell-Miller, H. (2019). HOMESIDE: A home-based family caregiver-delivered music intervention for people living with dementia: Protocol of a randomised controlled trial. *British Medical Journal Open.* https://doi.org/10.1136/bmjopen-2019-031332

Baker, F. A., Stretton-Smith, P., Sousa, T. A., Clark, I., Cotton, A., Gold, C., & Lee, Y.-E. C. (2020). Process and resource assessment in trials undertaken in residential care homes: Experiences from the Australian MIDDEL research team. *Contemporary Clinical Trials Communication.* https://doi.org/10.1016/j.conctc.2020.100675

Baker, F. A., Tamplin, J., Rickard, N., Ponsford, J., New, P., & Lee, Y.-E. C. (2019). A therapeutic songwriting intervention to promote reconstruction of self-concept and enhance wellbeing following brain and spinal cord injury: Pilot randomised controlled trial. *Clinical Rehabilitation.* https://doi.org/10.1177/0123456789123456. First Published 22 February 2019.

Belbin, M. (2010). *Team roles at work* (2nd ed.). Routledge.

Bourgault, A. M., & Goforth, C. (2021). Embrace teamwork to create and maintain a positive workplace culture. *Critical Care Nurse, 41*(3), 8–10. https://doi.org/10.4037/ccn2021662

Clark, I. N., Baker, F. A., Peiris, C. L., Shoebridge, G., & Taylor, N. F. (2016). Participant-selected music and physical activity in older adults following cardiac rehabilitation: A randomised controlled trial. *Clinical Rehabilitation.* https://doi.org/10.1177/0269215516640864. First published on line 6 April 2016.

Cook, S. (2009). *Building a high performance team: Proven techniques for effective team working.* IT Governance Pub.

Davies, R., Tamplin, J., Baker, F. A., Bajo, E., Bolger, K., Sheers, N., & Berlowitz, D. (2016). Music-assisted relaxation during transition to non-Invasive ventilation in people with Motor Neuron Disease: A qualitative case series. *British Journal of Music Therapy, 30*(2), 74–82. https://doi.org/10.1177/1359457516669153

Flight, L., Julious, S., Brennan, A., Todd, S., & Hind, D. (2020). How can health economics be used in the design and analysis of adaptive clinical trials? A qualitative analysis. *TRIALS, 21*(1), 252. https://doi.org/10.1186/s13063-020-4137-2

Loi, S. M., Flynn, L., Cadwallader, C., Stretton-Smith, P., Bryant, C., & Baker, F. A. (2022). Music and psychology and social connections program: Protocol for a novel intervention for dyads affected by younger-onset dementia. *Brain Sciences, 12*(4), 503. https://doi.org/10.3390/brainsci12040503

Makris, U. E., Ferrante, L. E., & Mody, L. (2018). Leadership lessons: Building and nurturing a high-performing clinical research team. *Journal of the American Geriatrics Society, 7*, 1258.

Polanco, F. R., Dominguez, D. C., Grady, C., Stoll, P., Ramos, C., Mican, J. M., Miranda-Acevedo, R., Morgan, M., Jeasmine, A., Purdie, L., & Rivera-Goba, M. V. (2011). Conducting HIV research in racial and ethnic minority communities: Building a successful interdisciplinary research team. *Journal of the Association of Nurses in AIDS Care, 22*(5), 388–396. https://doi.org/10.1016/j.jana.2010.10.008

Tamplin, J., Baker, F. A., Bolger, K., Bajo, E., Davies, R., Sheers, N., & Berlowitz, D. (2017). Exploring the feasibility of music-assisted relaxation intervention on the transition to non-invasive ventilation in people with Motor Neuron Disease. *Music Medicine, 19*(2), 86–97.

Tamplin, J., Morris, M., Marigliani, C., Baker, F. A., Noff, G., & Vogel, A. P. (2020). ParkinSong: Outcomes of a 12-month controlled trial of therapeutic singing groups in Parkinson's disease. *Journal of Parkinson's Disease.* https://doi.org/10.3233/JPD-191838

Thorn, J. C., Davies, C. F., Brookes, S. T., Noble, S. M., Dritsaki, M., Gray, E., Hughes, D. A., Mihaylova, B., Petrou, S., Ridyard, C., Sach, T., Wilson, E. C. F., Wordsworth, S., & Hollingworth, W. (2021). Content of health economics analysis plans (HEAPs) for trial-based economic evaluations: Expert Delphi consensus survey. *Value in Health, 24*(4), 539–547. https://doi.org/10.1016/j.jval.2020.10.002

Zapf, A., Rauch, G., & Kieser, M. (2020). Why do you need a biostatistician? *BMC Medical Research Methodology, 20*(1), 1–6. https://doi.org/10.1186/s12874-020-0916-4

CHAPTER 5

Budgeting for Success: Management and Resource Planning

BARRIERS AND ENABLERS TO EFFECTIVE RESOURCE MANAGEMENT

Clinical trials that are powered to detect a clinically significant change in health outcomes often attract high costs. Costs are driven by the time and resources needed to plan, manage, monitor, analyse, and report on all trial activities including governance, recruitment, intervention implementation, data collection, and statistical analysis (Bentley et al., 2019). Notably, the costs of implementing trials are increasing year by year, in part due to the increasing number and complexity of governance and regulatory approval processes that are needed to ensure the trial is safe, ethical, feasible, and will not lead to research waste[1] (Bentley et al., 2019; Hind et al., 2017). And while the costs are increasing, research budgets in many parts of the world are contracting, especially in the United States, Europe, and Canada (Chakma et al., 2014). This presents a challenge for all researchers trying to secure funding to implement a trial; creative arts therapy researchers are not exempt from these challenges. Further, we are competing for funds with hundreds of other researchers who all want to apply for the limited available funds to implement a scientifically sound

---

[1] Research waste is a term commonly used to describe the poor use of money and resources that have led to no useful outcomes. See Chapter 1 for a discussion on research waste.

study. We need to provide compelling arguments as to the scientific rigor of our projects, its benefit to end-users and society, while also presenting a realistic and competitive budget. We need to show value-for-money.

High costs of delivering trials can become a barrier for researchers as they might design a perfect study, only to discover that it is prohibitively expensive and that they are not able to have the trial adequately funded. Randomised controlled trials that involve a comparative intervention (control or other), usually need large number of participants to be sufficiently powered to detect intervention effects. Designated members of the research team need to be masked to allocation (this an exercise that takes careful planning) and then obtain data from multiple participants. Such processes are costly but necessary to generate non-biased findings that are trustworthy, compelling, and conclusive.

While we may be excellent creative arts therapy researchers, skills in budget estimation, planning, and monitoring may not be a skill set that we have had training for. Our doctoral education was more focused on ensuring we could become independent in designing and implementing research studies, and analysing the data generated by them. To date, I have yet to meet any creative arts therapy researcher who claims to have had training in budget management. Yet appropriate project budget estimates and prudent spending are needed and there seems to be an assumption by our administering organisations, that we possess competencies in this area.

The researcher is often presented with a maximum funding amount, so the project needs to be appropriately scaled to be achievable within this budget. This means the researcher needs a reasonable understanding of the scope and resources needed to implement the proposed study. A budget of US$50,000 does not go far when wanting to implement a randomised controlled trial. At best, a feasibility or pilot study could be achieved within that budget. When budgets increase to US$200,000–$500,000, a more sizeable and complex study can be planned and dependent upon the study design and anticipated effect size, might even be sufficiently resourced to implement an adequately powered study. And when budgets are at least US$1 million, researchers can plan to design high quality, complex, powered, impactful, and policy-influencing studies. But, as Hind et al. (2017) state, estimating the direct costs associated with study implementation, is "an inexact exercise".

For example, our MIDDEL study (Baker et al., 2022) which aimed to recruit 500 participants from 28 care homes and implement music interventions in each two to four times per week for 6 months. A significant component of our budget (US$318,000, 43% of the total budget) was devoted to implementing 6,500 45-minute interventions. This compares with the HOMESIDE (Baker et al., 2019) budget, with a comparable sample size of 495, only 990 2-hour intervention sessions were provided per dyad, the interventions cost approximately 15% of the total budget.[2]

There are several factors that make budget planning challenging including budgeting for the unknown—such as being in the middle of a research project during a worldwide pandemic where plans are forcibly interrupted by external forces. It is advisable to build in a little "fat" into your budget for such unforeseen events. For example, if a member of the research team decides to leave the project, recruiting and training a new person to deliver interventions or collect data will take time and resources. Similarly, delays in arranging research agreements with industry partners such as hospitals or schools, may mean the project is delayed. Any unexpected delays will impact the budget. Building in fat of around 15% is advisable if allowable.

One of the challenges of estimating resources needed for a project is that resources needed can fluctuate during the different phases of the project and can be dependent upon what types of activities are being undertaken at that time. As described later, there are a lot of tasks needing attention early in the trial development, prior to the first participant enrolment and therefore, resources needed at the beginning of the study are high. Once the study is up and running, there may be periods of time when resources needed are lower. A flexible budget can accommodate these peaks and troughs, for example, by using casual staff during known peak periods. Flexibility in employment contracts for some staff members during key periods can also be helpful. Hind et al. (2017) found that savings could be made when reducing the project manager from 100 to 40% during the recruitment period, and to 20% during the period when participants were being followed up. An example in my own study was how I managed the employment contract for the biostatistician. For HOMESIDE, the biostatistician was critical at the beginning of the trial

---

[2] There were differences in allocated funding for interventions in different countries dependent upon how research staffing was set-up and funding regulations in each country.

as the project was being set-up and randomisation processes were developed (20% for year 1). During the data collection period, there was less work needed, with the role focused more on developing the Statistical Analysis Plan (SAP) (see Chapter 9) and preparing reports for the Data Safety Monitoring Board (10% for years 2 and first half of years 3) (see Chapter 3). At the end of the data collection period, the biostatistician's role increased substantially as they finalised the SAP and proceeded with the analysis and interpretation of data (60% for the final 6-months).

The use of casual versus fixed-term staff does however raise some challenges. While casualisation of staffing allows for the principal investigator to have control over the budget to capitalise on peaks and reduce costs during troughs, in my experience, this is not always the best option to choose. Employing staff on fixed-term contracts (1 to 4 years), maximises investment as staff have more buy-in and ownership of the project, and therefore are more likely to give it their 100% commitment. Managing anticipated peaks and troughs can then be managed by ensuring "all hands are on deck" during anticipated peak times, and staff take planned paid leave (i.e. vacations) during trial periods where there is low activity. Additionally, if you are a principal investigator who has two or three concurrent medium to large size studies being implemented, you can be flexible with what tasks your staff participate in. If one project has a period of minimal activity, staff paid by that grant, can be asked to support staff working on a different project. Examples of this were in the MIDDEL (Baker et al., 2022) and MATCH studies, both projects being funded by the same funding body. While waiting for the biostatisticians to analyse the MIDDEL data, the rest of the research team had little tasks to do so they were temporarily reassigned to support the MATCH team who were in the midst of the busy start-up phase of the trial. Then, when the MIDDEL analysis was completed, they were redirected back to MIDDEL to support the write up of the main outcomes paper.

One of the most significant learnings for me over the past 5 years, is not to underestimate the time (and therefore costs) required to plan the project implementation. With the usual success rates for submitted grants being less than 20%, researchers often have a "submit, forget, and move on" attitude towards the grant submission process. Researchers cannot afford to wait in the hope their submission will be successful, instead, you just look out for the next potential opportunity. This is certainly my attitude, and one that protects me from being too disappointed when I receive the "unsuccessful" correspondence from the funding body.

However, when you do happen to be notified of winning a grant, it can take you by surprise. From that moment, the project "clock" is already on and the timeline to study completion already in situ. Therefore, and ideally, the "submit, forget, and move on" attitude should be tempered a little, with some project planning occurring in between the submission and expected awarded grant announcement dates.

Planning and start-up administrative costs associated with commencing new trials have been the predominant driver of increased clinical trial costs (Bentley et al., 2019). Resourcing governance requirements such as obtaining approvals from multiple institutional ethics review board (IRBs) (see Chapter 3) and contracts with study sites and project partners can be costly, not just in terms of fees, but the often-lengthy process can lead to delays in commencement of the study, thereby having an impact on project budget. Other tasks that take time but must be completed prior to implementation include writing the protocol, recruiting, and training staff, study site set-up, and set-up of the clinical trial database (Speich et al., 2020). The time and resources needed to plan a study from its conception until the first participant is enrolled is estimated at mean 192 days for a large RCT to 295 days for a multi-site RCT (Speich et al., 2019). When reflecting on my own trials, in all cases, the lead up time to enrolling the first participants was insufficient. For example, in the HOMESIDE clinical trial which had a leadership team of 6 (me as principal investigator, and a country leader in each of the five participating countries), we received notice of success in November 2018. Immediately, we set to work planning multi-institutional agreements, data sharing agreements, study protocol development, client report forms, ethics, and database development, and by the time we were ready to enrol our first participant, 11 months had passed. In our original plan, we anticipated enrolling our first participant at month 7. I offer some suggestions to reduce that length later in this chapter.

Leveraging from a researcher's existing networks and collaborating in various ways can improve efficiencies in trial delivery. One way to increase efficiencies in recruitment is to work closely with researchers from other trials where participant inclusion criteria is similar. For example, our HOMESIDE study recruited participant-carers and people living with dementia who were diagnosed with moderate to severe symptoms of dementia. We collaborated with the SHAPE study (Self-management and health promotion in early-stage dementia with e-learning for carers) who were working with people with dementia who were in much earlier states of disease progression. When we screened participants who were too early in the disease progression to be eligible for our study, we referred them to the SHAPE study. Similarly, the SHAPE research team referred people to the HOMESIDE study when their potential participants were assessed as too far progressed in their disease to be eligible for their study.

Preparing a Study Budget

Preparing the budget will require the chief investigator to estimate the amount of time in hours, weeks, and months needed to complete study tasks by personnel employed specifically for the project.[3] Although granting bodies may request higher level budgets, it can be helpful for the research team to have a more fine-grained budget that details a list of activities within the different phases of the trial. Once these are identified, the investigators can break these tasks down into their components and estimate the time, resources and overall costs associated with implementing them. The major components of the trial budget are:

1. Project design and set-up.
2. Ethics, contracts, and other regulatory processes.
3. Trial monitoring and quality assurance.
4. Trial master file handling and administration.
5. Data management.
6. Statistics, reports, and publication.
7. Project management.
8. Patient and public involvement.
9. Site costs.

Project Design and Set-Up

As mentioned earlier, the project planning stage can take a significant amount of time, especially for complex projects, and usually more than you anticipate. Perhaps the first task required is to develop staff position descriptions, advertise, interview, and recruit people who will work

---

[3] By this, I mean personnel such as post-doctoral researchers, project managers, data managers, clinicians, etc., that are not in continuing positions (tenured) within their universities. So, for example, my own time is not budgeted as this is considered an "in-kind" contribution to the project.

with the investigators on the project. Choosing the right people with the needed skill set, appropriate experience, and who are suitably qualified is an important first step. Depending upon your institution, you may need to include a budget for advertising. Once staff have been appointed and onboarding is completed, you and your team will need to progress the project set-up. These tasks include development of the full protocol, the intervention protocol and fidelity checklists, and risk assessment plan, and drafting the plain language statements, informed consent forms and other project materials such as leaflets and questionnaires (and translating them to other languages when relevant). The research team needs to develop client report forms, and checklists needed for study site visits, and build and test the database. The investigators will then provide staff training on the study procedures, and pilot recruitment approaches, data collection, intervention delivery, and data entry to check for possible omissions, errors, and procedures that require clarity and anything else that will help avoid or mitigate challenges further down the track.

I mentioned earlier that for our HOMESIDE trial, it took us 11 months to complete the planning stage, however, this time could have been reduced if we had employed our research staff earlier. Prior to their appointment, the investigators were the only ones involved in planning, and we were balancing these tasks alongside our teaching and other university responsibilities. Once the project team were appointed, the time between their onboarding and enrolment of the first participant was 7 months. The main point here is, that the time between commencement of the project and first enrolled participant is dependent upon how much available time the investigators have to plan the project, how many hours their project staff are employed to support these activities, and how skilled (and independent) they are in completing the required tasks. When developing the budget for staffing, consider adding a margin of 15%, to accommodate wage rises, unforeseen delays and extra capacity needs during the study.

In addition to the staffing costs during start-up, there may be costs related to regulatory processes such as ethics committees, legal costs associated with developing multi-institutional agreements, or insurance (see Chapter 3). The cost of trial insurance may be high for some trials, dependent upon the risk associated with the project implementation. Insurance requirements are likely to be quite different in the public health sector compared with the private and are likely to differ between countries.

Project Implementation

Models to Budget for Recruitment

One of the most resource intensive components of clinical trials is recruitment. In our own MIDDEL study, we evaluated the time required to recruit 318 participants from a total of 666 individuals screened (Baker et al., 2020) (see Chapter 6). Recruitment involves first identifying participants (whether they self-refer or their names are provided to the research team via a gatekeeper), making contact to explain the study, screening for eligibility, and then obtaining informed consent. Dependent upon context, population being recruited, and the potential total number of eligible participants, this can be a long and tedious process for research teams. Each component of the recruitment process can be costed—preparation of materials, advertising, training of recruitment staff, management of recruitment data, staff contact time with participants, and participant incentives. In our MIDDEL study, we had little difficulty identifying participants as they were all residents of very large residential aged care facilities, however, time and resources were needed in contacting next of kin, explaining the study and obtaining informed consent (see Baker et al., 2020). In HOMESIDE, we had the reverse issue, obtaining informed consent was relatively quick and easy but we did have long and lengthy processes in terms of reaching potential participants. For example, for the Australian team, 50% of the clinical trial manager's time was spent on recruitment (2½ days per week) including screening participants, reaching out to referring organisations, drafting advertisements, etc.

There are two models a researcher can use to fund recruitment activities. The first is known as a cost-reimbursement model (Lovegreen et al., 2018) which would typically cover costs for personnel time. This could be members of the research team who are employees of the university or researching institution, or they could be subcontractors of the sites where the study is being implemented. For example, a nurse or administration person employed by a hospital engages in recruitment tasks on behalf of the research team, and the institution invoices the university for the hours spent on that work. This model has some disadvantages as there is no incentive to recruit quickly, leading to slow or underperformance and subsequently a large proportion of the budget is used to recruit, reducing the budget available for funding the remaining components of the trial.

The second approach is known as the "performance-based only" model (Lovegreen et al., 2018). Here, the researchers outsource the recruitment process to either the site or an external contractor to recruit on a predetermined reimbursement amount per participant. This approach can be very efficient because it can reduce expenditure during slow recruitment, and, more importantly, is results-oriented. Therefore, it rewards performance, thereby increasing engagement and effort on the part of the recruiter. One does need to be mindful, however, that the recruiter maintains good ethical practice and that there is no participant coercion, due to the incentive model that performance-based reimbursement attracts.

Licensing Fees

During the study implementation period, the team may need to allocate funding for a range of licensing fees. These fees may include a per-person cost to use copyrighted questionnaires such as the Hospital Anxiety and Depression Scale (Zigmond & Snaith, 1983). In the case of dance/movement therapy or music therapy, there may also be costs associated with music licensing. For example, in testing our MATCH app, we needed to include a budget for a Spotify account for each person enrolled in the trial. This was at a cost of AUS$12 per month per participant.

Using Routinely Collected Data

Administering questionnaires and other outcome measures can be a costly component of clinical trials, especially when assessors need to be masked to allocation. Nevens et al. (2019) argue that researchers can make trials more efficient and less expensive when routinely collected data in registries or electronic health records are used instead of collecting new data specifically for the purposes of the research. In our MIDDEL study, we did exactly this. Firstly, we used electronic data systems at some of the residential aged care homes to track incidences of PRN medication use, agitation, and adverse events, and we also contracted the national MEDICARE Medical Benefits Scheme to collate data on doctor and other healthcare visits, hospital admissions, and medication use for a per-participant fee. This was a more economical approach than paying a member of the research team to sit and painstakingly audit every patient file to extract the relevant data. Not only is this use of electronic data more efficient, but it also minimises the risk of data errors when transferring data from hard copy files into the electronic data capture system. It also ensures that the data set is complete and that there is no missing data.

Trial Site Visits and Monitoring

While every trial may have different monitoring needs, it is important to budget for staff time and direct costs associated with the initial visit and ongoing visits to study sites by the research team. Regular site visits by the project manager and principal investigator for monitoring can ensure that any deviations from the protocol are identified early. Similarly, site visits can be helpful in maintaining relationships with staff at the study site. The budget should include an allocation of time for preparation, travel, and reporting. To make monitoring more efficient, any opportunities for remote monitoring should be included (Nevens et al., 2019).

Governance Costs

There are a range of potential costs associated with governance. Budget allocations to fund the operations of the Data Safety Monitoring Board and/or advisory board may be necessary. This includes providing a "sitting fee" payment for each member who attends the meeting. This could cover their time for attending and preparing for the meeting and parking/travel costs. For the research team, there is considerable time needed to plan the meeting, develop and coordinate distribution of agendas and associated pre-meeting reading material, recording meeting actions, and distributing meeting minutes. In addition, the meetings might require a statistical analysis report to be developed and produced, again this requires time (and therefore can be costed). When allocating costs for governance, it can be helpful to estimate a cost per meeting.

Data Management and Analysis

The budget associated with data management needs to include the cost of designing and hosting the electronic database, importation of data into the database, monitoring for missing data and data quality, generating regular interim data reports, and eventually the database lock. Nevens et al. (2019) propose that dependent upon the trial complexity and duration, the data manager is likely to need between two and four hours of time per participant for data coding, programming queries, following-up on queries and resolving them. I have always communicated to my team that poorly collected and unreliable data is as bad as missing data (if not worse) so it is important that the data collected is monitored closely so any problems can be identified and resolved quickly. In our HOMESIDE trial, our data manager generated quarterly reports for each of the country lead investigators. It directed country leaders to follow-up with their relevant staff members on data missing or possible errors associated with certain participants. An experienced and senior member of the team is needed to lead the data management process and therefore appropriately funded staff time should be allocated for this.

Collecting and inputting data into a database is also an extremely time-consuming task and can take up a significant proportion of your budget. Therefore, when designing the trial, researchers should only collect the data needed to answer their research questions. There is always a danger that investigators are initially over-enthusiastic and want to collect data that cover many areas, purely because they are interesting, or collect qualitative data within mixed methods trials that is overly excessive. We made this error in HOMESIDE. The research team were eager to collect qualitative data that could be used as explanatory data to support the quantitative findings. We included diaries and interviews for every participant in the music and reading interventions. That was 330 diaries and 330 interviews. The diaries were necessary as we were capturing adherence, but the 330 interviews were perhaps a little excessive. Each interview required us to budget for a staff member to run the interview (2 hours), then transcribe the interview (5–8 hours), and then for a more senior member of the team to analyse the interviews (approximately 5–6 hours). That's a commitment of 16 hours per interview, or 5,280 hours. In other words, a lot of money! When considering most qualitative studies include less than 20 participants, 330 was unnecessary and unresourceful.

To make the process of data management and monitoring as efficient as possible, it can sometimes be helpful (if pragmatic and appropriate), to collect data and input it into the database at the same time, rather than collecting it on paper and later transferring it to the database. Many electronic databases such as REDCap (see Chapter 7), now have mobile applications which means the research staff can directly access and input the data into the database from anywhere, including patient hospital rooms when required. This not only represents a cost-saving to the project, but also limits the amounts of missing data, errors made while transferring data from paper into the database and is more secure than having some data collected on paper.

Finally, the budget should include costs associated with the development of the Statistical Analysis Plan, randomisation plan, and drafting of the statistical analysis and trial reports, and publications. Most funding bodies now require the main trial results to be published in freely accessible, open access journals. Journals do charge for this and therefore, publication fees should be a line item in your budget.

Project Management

As described in Chapter 4, the project manager is the key personnel to employ in a trial and appointing someone experienced and well qualified is a worthy investment. In addition to the salary of the project manager, there are many other direct costs associated with project management. These may include the costs associated with Trial Steering Committee meetings and investigator meetings including travel, accommodation, meals, etc., when investigators are not all located in the same city. These types of costs are often overlooked (Speich et al., 2020). While the COVID-19 pandemic has made us all adept at using online meetings, I still argue without reservation, that in-person meetings should be held when possible. Having experienced online meetings for the two middle years of the four-year HOMESIDE project, and soon after, the hybrid model, I can honestly say that nothing replaces the effectiveness of an in-person meetings when it comes to making important decisions.

Public and Patient Involvement and Public Engagement

Most granting bodies require trials to include public and patient involvement (PPI) (see Chapter 3). PPI committee members, once appointed, are asked to contribute to the work of the trial sometimes on an "as needed basis" or are asked to engage in regularly scheduled meetings. Appropriately remunerating these members including a sitting fee, provision of refreshments, and transport or parking reimbursement, should be added to the trial budget. Such remuneration is needed to ensure they feel valued and have project buy-in.

Knowledge Translation and Exchange, Public Engagement, and Advocacy

All projects need to have a knowledge translation and exchange plan (Chapter 10) including public engagement and advocacy. Dissemination can take the form of academic and non-academic publications, conference presentations, speaking at public events, social media announcements, and developing accessible mediums such as the production of short movies for YouTube, etc. These activities all come at a cost and should be budgeted during the planning phase of the trial. For example, open access fees for publishing the main findings can be costly with fees in 2022 in excess of US$5,000 in some of the top ranked journals. Costs for attending conferences should also be considered a priority for grant submissions. After all, what is the point in generating impactful findings when the plan to disseminate these findings is not appropriately budgeted for. Public events such as a project launch and project end celebrations can be means of disseminating project updates and findings to stakeholders and consumers. Costing in venue hire, refreshments, technology support, advertising, and event administration is needed.

Conclusion

Appropriately resourcing a project is important to ensure that sufficient funds are available to conduct all the activities needed to complete it. No matter how much you plan, unexpected expenses inevitably arise, and the principal investigator may be forced to make choices in how a fixed budget is used. Wherever possible, have extra "fat" in the budget to accommodate unexpected events and think carefully about which tasks may need to be conducted by the researchers in tenured positions rather than those employed solely by the project's budget. This will help in appropriately allocating budget to activities that should not/cannot be performed by the researchers who are not directly employed by a grant.

References

Baker, F. A., Bloska, J., Stensæth, K., Wosch, T., Bukowska, A., Braat, S., Sousa, T., Tamplin, J., Clark, I. N., Lee, Y.-E. C., Clarke, P., Lautenschlager, N., & Odell-Miller, H. (2019). HOMESIDE: A home-based family caregiver-delivered music intervention for people living with dementia: Protocol of a randomised controlled trial. *British Medical Journal Open.* https://doi.org/10.1136/bmjopen-2019-031332

Baker, F. A., Lee, Y.-E. C., Sousa, T. V., Stretton-Smith, P. A., Tamplin, J., Sveinsdottir, V., Geretsegger, M., Wake, J. D., Assmus, J., & Gold, C. (2022). Clinical effectiveness of Music Interventions for Dementia and

Depression in Elderly care (MIDDEL) in the Australian cohort: pragmatic cluster-randomised controlled trial. *The Lancet Healthy Longevity, 3*(3), e153–e165.

Baker, F. A., Stretton-Smith, P., Sousa, T. A., Clark, I., Cotton, A., Gold, C., & Lee, Y.-E. C. (2020). Process and resource assessment in trials undertaken in residential care homes: Experiences from the Australian MIDDEL research team. *Contemporary Clinical Trials Communication.* https://doi.org/10.1016/j.conctc.2020.100675

Bentley, C., Cressman, S., van der Hoek, K., Arts, K., Dancey, J., & Peacock, S. (2019). Conducting clinical trials—Costs, impacts, and the value of clinical trials networks: A scoping review. *Clinical Trials, 16*(2), 183–193. https://doi.org/10.1177/1740774518820060

Chakma, J., Sun, G. H., Steinberg, J. D., Sammut, S. M., & Jagsi, R. (2014). Asia's ascent—Global trends in biomedical R&D expenditures. *New England Journal of Medicine, 370*, 3–6.

Hind, D., Reeves, B., Bathers, S., Bray, C., Corkhill, A., Hayward, C., Harper, L., Napp, V., Norrie, J., Speed, C., Tremain, L., Keat, N., & Bradburn, M. (2017). Comparative costs and activity from a sample of UK clinical trial units. *Trials, 18*, 203. https://doi.org/10.1186/s13063-017-1934-3

Lovegreen, O., Riggs, D., Staten, M. A., Sheehan, P., & Pittas, A. G. (2018). Financial management of large, multi-center trials in a challenging funding milieu. *Trials, 19*(1), 267. https://doi.org/10.1186/s13063-018-2638-z

Nevens, H., Harrison, J., Vrijens, F., Verleye, L., Stocquart, N., Marynen, E., & Hulstaert, F. (2019). Budgeting of non-commercial clinical trials: Development of a budget tool by a public funding agency. *Trials, 20*(1), 1–10. https://doi.org/10.1186/s13063-019-3900-8

Speich, B., Gloy, V., Schur, N., Ewald, H., Hemkens, L. G., Schwenkglenks, M., & Briel, M. (2020). A scoping review shows that several nonvalidated budget planning tools for randomized trials are available. *Journal of Clinical Epidemiology, 117*, 9–19. https://doi.org/10.1016/j.jclinepi.2019.09.009

Speich, B., Schur, N., Gryaznov, D., von Niederhausern, B., Hemkens, L. G., Schandelmaier, S., Amstutz, A., Kasenda, B., Pauli-Magnus, C., Ojeda-Ruiz, E., Tomonaga, Y., McCord, K., Nordmann, A., von Elm, E., Briel, M., & Schwenkglenks, M. (2019). Resource use, costs, and approval times for planning and preparing a randomized clinical trial before and after the implementation of the new Swiss human research legislation. *PLoS ONE, 14*, e0210669.

Zigmond, A., & Snaith, R. (1983). The hospital anxiety and depression scale. *Acta Psychiatrica Scandinavica, 67*(6), 361–370. https://doi.org/10.1111/j.1600-0447.1983.tb09716.x

CHAPTER 6

Recruitment, Retention, and Follow-Up: Frustration or Bliss

INTRODUCTION

Participant recruitment and retention is a key component of every clinical trial. In an efficacy or effectiveness trial, once the required targeted sample size has been calculated, every effort must be made to reach that target sample, otherwise the trial will be considered "underpowered". Many planned trials are at the outset underpowered often because recruiting smaller sample sizes takes less time and reduced effort, and ultimately costs less. However, underpowered trials produce inconclusive data and increase the risk of not detecting a difference where a difference does exist (Type II error). Implementing an underpowered trial might be regarded as "research waste". Research waste refers to the wasted time, energy, and funding to produce research that (a) may not answer high-priority questions, (b) employs poor designs, (c) is never published because researchers do not wish to report "disappointing" results, or (d) does not report all planned outcomes (Chalmers & Glasziou, 2009). A movement to reduce and avoid research waste is gaining momentum at present (Gardner, 2018), with the argument that "we need less research, better research, and research done for the right reasons" (Altman, 1994). In the context of recruitment and retention of participants, the trial might be regarded as wasteful if it fails to reach the sample needed to answer high-priority questions. We have an ethical obligation not to waste participants' time who voluntarily participate in a study based on a belief the trial will contribute to healthcare knowledge and practice. Often in good faith, they enrol in the trial knowing the intervention could be potentially beneficial but equally potentially harmful for the sole purpose of assisting the researchers to generate statistically meaningful findings. It requires a commitment in time, effort, and at times discomfort, so if we enrol people into trials, we have a responsibility to design a trial that is sufficiently powered to answer the posed research questions.

Achieving the target sample size is a major concern of all research teams when it comes to managing a clinical trial—and it is certainly the component of the trial that attracts much of my attention and energy during the planning and operational phases of the trial. A recent Cochrane review found a staggering 44% of trials unsuccessfully reached their target sample size (Treweek et al., 2018). Many studies will employ recruitment strategies that are implemented in an ad hoc manner, and certainly during my early years in clinical research, that was my approach. Adopting ad hoc approaches and later comparing recruitment strategies retrospectively and observationally to determine what were most or least successful strategies are inefficient and can be very resource intensive. Researchers have recognised this challenge and note that there is an increasing trend in clinical trial research to employ the use of a "study within a trial" (SWAT) method. These "sub-studies" aim to assess the impact of trial design innovations (such as a recruitment approach) on a trial's efficiency (Treweek et al., 2018). Later in this chapter, I outline a range of recruitment strategies that have been systematically reviewed, but at this early point in the chapter, it is important to note that every study is unique in its design, research questions, the population under investigation, and the context within which the research is being implemented, and as such, recruitment strategies need to be tailored to each specific trial. In other words, this chapter offers ideas and strategies that have been used in my own studies as well as other published studies, but each researcher will need to design (and pilot) their own recruitment methods to suit their own study.

The reasons why such a large proportion of studies fail to reach their sample size, is complex. At the most obvious level, there may be too few potential eligible participants available to recruit that the research team has access too. This scenario occurred during my first ever pilot randomised controlled trial of people who had acquired aphasia following a stroke, where I was piloting a novel intervention known as Melodic Intonation Therapy (Baker, 2011). Based on retrospective data made available to me, I estimated that there would be enough potential participants who had a diagnosis of post-stroke aphasia over a 3-year period to reach my sample. I only needed a sample size of 15 for the pilot, something that seemed achievable at the time. However, my error was that I had stipulated such tight eligibility criteria, that over the three years, only four met the inclusion criteria. There are two lessons I learned from this experience. First, it is important to estimate the potential pool of participants based on the "actual" inclusion criteria rather than just basing it on a more general diagnostic category, and second, consider ensuring that eligibility criteria are more inclusive (and representative) of the population.

A converse scenario of why trials may not reach their target sample size could be that there are not enough "consenting" participants. A trial may have access to large numbers of eligible participants, but for any number of reasons, the uptake and/or retention of participants may be low. I experienced this in scenario in one of my randomised controlled trial of people with spinal cord injury and brain injury. The study was testing the effects of an innovative songwriting program that focused on exploring identity post-injury (Baker, Tamplin, et al., 2019). We had calculated a target sample size of 64 participants (2-arm study, 32 participants per arm), but only reached a sample size of 47. Before commencing the trial, we knew there would be sufficient potential participants meeting our inclusion criteria, however, what we had not anticipated, was that a significant proportion of participants declined to participate. After screening 1,153 patients and excluding those who were not contactable, we had identified and approached 246 eligible participants. Of these, 189 (77%) declined to participate. Reasons for not consenting fell into one main category—timing. Timing related firstly to their perceived need to focus solely on their physical rehabilitation program, and they did not want any potential distractions, or secondly, because they felt they were not in the right emotional state to be confronted with their situation; they were in survival mode at that time. These are perhaps logical decisions a person might take when deciding whether to take part in a trial. Our error was that we did not explore fully, the potential uptake of the study when estimating the resources and time needed to recruit our full sample. These reasons to decline trial participation and others will be explored more fully in this chapter, along with strategies to mitigate these.

Why Do People Choose to Participate in Research?

To increase the chances of enrolling "consenting" participants, it is helpful in every research context to understand why people might accept or decline study participation. Once the research team has this knowledge, they can devise a recruitment strategy that takes these reasons into consideration. People choose to take up opportunities to participate in research from one of two broad reasons. The first relates to their personal belief that they will benefit from the research, and the second is for altruistic reasons that they want to contribute to the advancement of healthcare (Gardner, 2018).

First and foremost, people consent because they have the perceived belief that the proposed intervention will improve their health. Dependent upon the diagnosis or prognosis, people may volunteer to be part of new novel treatments in the hope of better health or a better quality of life, or quicker access to healthcare than they might receive when there may be waiting lists for some health services. There is a sense of safety and reassurance through the close and regular monitoring they may receive from the research team; extra support than they might receive otherwise (Natale et al., 2021). Further, when people who are from lower socioeconomic backgrounds (from contexts where healthcare is a fee-for-service arrangement) are offered the opportunity to participate, they view this as an opportunity for "free healthcare" that they might not otherwise be able to afford.

While motivation to participate might stem from belief in the potential for better health outcomes, the notion of clinical equipoise can make this troublesome for those recruiting participants. Equipoise is a state of genuine uncertainty on the part of the research team regarding the effectiveness of the intervention under investigation (Cook & Sheets, 2011). When approaching potential participants, the recruiting team member wants to convey an unbiased perspective, but faced with participants who are searching for possible solutions to their health problems. There is a fine balance between conveying the research in a way that is attractive to participants but at the same time not risking therapeutic misconception (Lidz & Appelbaum, 2002).

The second reason people may participate in research is for altruistic reasons. People want to participate in trials to help future generations who may be affected by the same conditions (Naidoo et al., 2020). There is a sense that participation in research is contributing to the "common good"

(Natale et al., 2021). Some participants recognise that they have been the beneficiaries of earlier people's willingness to participate in trials, and this is their opportunity to give back and do the same for the generations to come (Bonevski et al., 2014; Natale et al., 2021). As one of our study participants said once "paying it forward".

WHY DO PEOPLE DECLINE PARTICIPATION IN RESEARCH?

There is a whole plethora of reasons why people choose to decline invitations to participate in research. Some stem from participant factors such as language barriers that impact their ability to understand the research study, concern for negative health effects, fears related to stigma, concern for psychological and physical burden, and the financial and personal costs of participation. Other reasons include lack of recruiter enthusiasm, gatekeeper pathways and discouragement from family members.

Health Status and Stigma

Some participants are reluctant to engage in research when they feel that their condition is being well managed, and they therefore decline to participate in a trial to maintain their status quo. Participants might have their condition under control but don't want to risk decline in health by trying something else. Conversely, other participants may already feel overwhelmed by their health condition or disease, and therefore when presented with opportunities to participate in research, they are not in the right mental state to cope with any additional information (Natale et al., 2021). This scenario was already highlighted earlier when participants in our neurodisability study (Baker, Tamplin, et al., 2019), felt too emotionally vulnerable to engage in a therapy that may temporarily emotionally destabilise them and potentially lower their motivation to participate in an active rehabilitation program. Additionally, the instability of a person's health status might influence their decision not to participate. For example, if a health condition is chronic and fluctuating in severity, they might fear that they are unable to commit to the project (e.g. if there is a risk of hospitalisation) (Forsat et al., 2020).

Co-morbidities may mean some people are ineligible to participate. To maximise the recruitment activities, it is important to develop your inclusion criteria so that you only exclude co-morbidities that may directly influence the treatment outcome. To give one example, in our residential aged care music intervention study (Baker et al., 2022; Gold et al., 2019), we were examining the impact of music on depression. We excluded people with significant hearing loss that could not be managed with hearing aids because for obvious reasons, this was a study about the impact of music interventions. At the same time, we allowed for co-morbidities such as anxiety.

While society has moved forward considerably with respect to an inclusive perspective on people with varying health conditions, some people would argue that stigma may still influence people's willingness to participate in research. Because of the stigma around certain health conditions (for example mental health), is still present, many people with those underlying conditions may choose to keep silent, not reveal their health status to others, and consequently decline invitations to participate (Brown et al., 2014).

Scepticism, Fear and Mistrust

Research has demonstrated that some participants do not sign up for studies because there is a general feeling of scepticism, fear, and mistrust in the research process (Natale et al., 2021). While ethics committees have made it mandatory to clearly explain how personal data will be used in studies, all of which is documented in the plain language statement, some participants still express concern about potential breach of confidentiality and access to their personal data, and how their data will be used (Baker et al., 2020; Natale et al., 2021). One example of this fear was highlighted by Brown et al. (2014) who suggested that recent immigrants who had not yet received permanent residency feared their data about their health status may be reported to authorities and place them at risk of deportation. Some potential participants are concerned about being treated like a "guinea pig" for interventions that are not yet approved for general use (Natale et al., 2021) or that the research is only being used to further the career of the researcher (Naidoo et al., 2020). This fear of having health professionals taking advantage of them was widespread, particularly from minority groups (Natale et al., 2021).

Mistrust is particularly apparent in some cultural groups such as African Americans, Hispanic-Americans, South Asian heritage, and Indigenous populations who have had a history of being mistreated or exploited in medical research and are less trusting of medical professionals (Bonevski et al., 2014; Brown et al., 2014; Forsat et al., 2020). Many studies implemented in Western developed countries have samples with an over-representation of white, middle class, highly educated people, and an under-representation of those from socially disadvantaged groups (NIH, 2004) for these very reasons. Our own Australian research with people living with dementia had low levels of participation by many ethnic minorities, despite intentionally selecting residential aged care homes with higher numbers of non-English speaking residents (Lee et al., 2022). An absence of data representing diversity in the population may limit the generalisability of the findings and threaten external validity of the study. Without data of a more diverse sample, the benefits and safety of health interventions cannot be guaranteed for those populations who are not represented in the sample. Researchers should take measures to address this challenge and adequately resource that aspect of recruitment accordingly (Bonevski et al., 2014).

Addressing trust has been thought to increase recruitment rates (Masood et al., 2019). Trust is a complex multidimensional concept that is based on expectations of respect and fidelity, competence, transparency, and confidentiality (Ahmed et al., 2019). Researchers need to be aware that trust should not be implicitly assumed but needs to be fostered and earned (McDonald et al., 2008). When researchers approach ethnic groups to purposefully engage them in research, the first goal should be to enable those in the group to feel empowered to voice their opinions about the research and for the researcher to gain an insider perspective. Without this, the researcher will not be able to adapt the research tools, methods, and interventions to ensure they are culturally appropriate and sensitive (Bonevski et al., 2014).

Engaging support from community groups and getting to know the community in a non-research environment can help to address mistrust, fear of research, and concurrently limit any existing gatekeeper blocks to recruitment (Ahmed et al., 2019; Bonevski et al., 2014). This pre-clinical trial engagement is particularly helpful when working with communities where there are hierarchical structures. An excellent example of this is the Australian Aboriginal communities whose elders provide leadership and guidance to younger members of the community. Having buy-in from these elders will aid recruitment.

Family Factors

The family context and influences of family members can shape a person's decision to participate in a research study. Families play a role in whether a participant will sign up for a study. For example, male spouses/partners may disapprove of their partner's wish to participate and in cultures where women accept such submissive roles, they will comply (Brown et al., 2014). Another factor might be that parents of young children or grandparents of young children may have caring obligations that preclude them from participation (Brown et al., 2014).

In some studies, such as those focused on families, where consent is needed from two or more members of the family unit, participation is dependent all parties signing the consent form (Song et al., 2021). This can pose problems when one or more of the family members decline while others wish to participate. In our HOMESIDE clinical trial (Baker et al., 2019), a family carer and a person living with dementia were both study participants and must participate as a dyad. There have been several instances when the person living with dementia has decided they do not want to participate, sometimes for reasons related to time and burden, and at other times because the person is still grappling with the dementia diagnosis and is not emotionally ready to participate. In other cases, the carer declines to participate, also for reasons of burden and time limitations or because they have yet to emotionally process the dementia diagnosis. Researchers would benefit on being sensitive to the whole family context as there may be familial factors at play that lead to a decision to decline study participation.

Language Barriers

Informed consent means that the participant fully understands what the research is about, what will happen to them, what the risks are, what they are expected to do, and how their data will be used. When the research team does not share the same first language as the participant, participants might have difficulty understanding the information needed to arrive at a decision (Baker et al., 2020). When study details are unnecessarily lengthy and complex, and when the material is not written in their native language, participants fear signing up for something that they do not fully understand (Bonevski et al., 2014; Brown et al., 2014; Forsat et al., 2020). Some studies have utilised interpreters (Raven-Gregg et al., 2021) or enlisted the help of family members to break down and translate the study details so it is understandable to participants (Natale et al., 2021). Several systematic reviews report of studies conducted in the United States, found that recruitment increased when Spanish-speaking workers were engaged in the recruitment process (Bonevski et al., 2014; Brown et al., 2014; Masood et al., 2019).

Participant Burden

The level of real and imagined burden associated with study participation may be a major deterrent in a person's decision to enrol in a study (Naidoo et al., 2020). People may already be experiencing burden associated with managing their illness, so any request to add to this existing burden may not be well received. Participation may have an anticipated psychological impact, financial impact, or time impact or any combination of these, which affects their decision to enrol and complete trial participation.

Participation in a trial attracts a varied array of psychological burdens. Naidoo et al. (2020) suggest that participants experience stress when trying to understand the aims of the research, what they will be expected to do, and may become overwhelmed by the quantity of information presented to them. They may experience a sense of intimidation and confusion when presented with information that may use complex technical terms. The process of randomisation can also be something that can be a source of anxiety. For example, participants have expressed disappointment, anger, and depression when informed that they were allocated to the control arm; there was a sense of having missed out on the optimal treatment and, therefore, felt there was no benefit for them in participating in the research at all (Naidoo et al., 2020). One participant expressed that there was "… no hope for me…extremely depressed …went home and cried. To leave the hospital after an hour of filling forms … empty handed. I felt no one really understood how bad I felt". Others have described it as like being in a lottery or Russian roulette (Natale et al., 2021) which suggests they were uncomfortable with their lack of control over an outcome that directly affects them. It is important to remember that due to various health challenges, they may already be experiencing a sense of being out of control, and a lack of choice of treatment arm could exacerbate that feeling (Brown et al., 2014).

Some participants have expressed psychological stress when they felt pressured to make a quick decision of whether to consent to participate. Some studies may be time critical—for example when working with people who are emerging from coma after receiving a brain injury. In my first ever study of people who were in post-traumatic amnesia (Baker, 2001), I needed to study people who were in this phase of recovery from acquired brain injury, over three consecutive days. This phase in their recovery may only last three to four days, so time was of the essence, otherwise they would no longer be eligible to participate. Families were approached inviting them to consent at a time when their loved one's health status was rapidly changing. An experienced member of the hospital staff was assigned to recruit and was very sensitive and conscious to minimise psychological burden. Some families did want more time to consider the study and respectively declined participation.

Engagement in a clinical trial may involve a commitment to attend a therapy program (sometimes over many weeks and months), engage in testing over multiple occasions, or responding to daily text messages asking participants to respond to questions about their health status, mood, or other important data (Baker et al., 2020). And despite researchers' efforts to minimise burden of engagement, some trial activities unavoidably expect a lot of participants to assess the real impact of an intervention. For example, in our HOMESIDE randomised controlled trial (Baker et al., 2019), we expected our participants to commit 45 hours of engagement in trial activities over 6-months comprising the following:

- Participate in completing an initial assessment: 2 hours.
- Participate in three online music or reading training sessions (intervention arms): total 4 hours
- Discuss intervention use with research team via 15-minute fortnightly phone calls over 12 weeks: 1½ hours
- Use music and reading as a therapy with the person they are caring for 5 times per week, for 30 minutes, for 12 weeks: 30 hours
- Complete short diary questions 5 times per week for 12 weeks, for 5 minutes: 5 hours
- Complete post-intervention assessments at 13 weeks and 26 weeks at 60 minutes each: 2 hours
- Complete a semi-structured interview post intervention: 1 hour.

It was evident that some participants declined because the engagement was perceived as too burdensome for them. Brown et al. (2014) found that lack of time was cited in studies conducted in the United States as the most common reason for Latinos to decline, and this was evidenced across all age groups. Participants sometimes report that researchers mistakably assumed that they had endless amounts of time available to participate in the research (Naidoo et al., 2020). Further, participants may have other competing commitments scheduled at the same time as the proposed research activities, particularly with respect to family and employment responsibilities (Dunleavy et al., 2018). Participating in the research may have forced them to make a choice between picking up children from school or trying to get on top of an ever-growing list of day-to-day commitments (Brown et al., 2014). Similarly, there were logistical challenges such as travel to certain sites for data collection. Travel was sometimes viewed as an inconvenient timewaster, especially if participants were randomised into the standard care arm of the trial and were not deriving any personal benefit from participation.

Another deterrent to participation might relate to financial burdens associated with participation. Costs might include travel costs such as parking or taxi fares, the costs of childminding, or the loss of income associated with needing to make appointments during normal business hours (Brown et al., 2014). The participant may need to weigh up the benefit of participation with the financial outlay or income loss.

Developing and Monitoring the Recruitment Strategy

After 20 years as a researcher, I have begun to appreciate the need for a carefully devised and monitored recruitment strategy. Social marketing (UyBico et al., 2007) has been increasingly utilised for the past two decades to influence behaviour and improve the welfare of society (Teemil, 2019) and has been identified as a suitable framework to organise and plan recruitment activities including studies of carers of people with dementia (Nichols et al., 2004) and of people in palliative care (LeBlanc et al., 2013). The aspects of social marketing framework that are relevant to study recruitment are participants, product, study promotion, price, and partners (Dunleavy et al., 2018).

Participants

The first step in developing the recruitment strategy is to identify where your potential participants can be sourced from. This might involve a bit of informal "market research" such as discussing with the members of your patient and public involvement (PPI) committee (consumers) and stakeholders, where you may be most likely to have direct contact with potential participants or gatekeepers. It might be helpful to start with what might be termed "low-lying fruit". These are places where you are likely to be given access to high numbers of the target participant group. Some examples of low-lying fruit may be to employ a professional recruitment company, approach professional networks, databases of potential participants that are either publicly available, or where you can be given access to a database of potential participants via a gatekeeper who is supportive of your research. Once you have exploited the low-lying fruit, you can begin to develop other recruitment strategies as described later in this chapter.

Developing the Research Promotional Product

The promotional materials that you develop to attract interest in study participation can be the make or break of your recruitment strategy. Therefore, investing time in developing, testing, and revising the material is essential, and it can take time to get it right. The product must be engaging enough to attract attention, socially and culturally acceptable, and provide adequate information that will enable a potential applicant (or gatekeeper) to determine whether participation might be of interest to them. At the same time, the promotional materials should not be overly detailed that it might scare off potential interest. Keep it simple and succinct to minimise the possibility of misunderstanding and try to keep the more relevant information at the forefront. These strategies will address language barriers for those with low literacy levels.

> *Case Study. Development of HOMESIDE Recruitment Materials.* In our HOMESIDE study, we developed various promotional materials including a recruitment video, flyers, posters, and scripts for radio interviews. We approached our PPI committee members and asked them to review our designs and bring a user perspective into the co-design of the promotional

> materials. We asked for input on language to check it was comprehendible, non-judgemental, and non-threatening (Crocker et al., 2015). They reviewed our original flyer and provided feedback that the colours of pale pink were not eye catching enough for older people, and white colour print does not stand out against the pink backgrounds. They felt that blue was a better colour, a soft blue "but not so soft that it would not be sufficiently contrasted with the white font". They also suggested bold colours that allowed a strong contrast between text and background is preferable for people living with dementia. Further recommendations included having lots of white space, information presented in point form, and including a QR code that links directly to the study website and webpage where people can register their interest to participate. They also noted that it needed to be more inclusive and explicitly invite people living with dementia in addition to their careers. They advised highlighting that joining the project was free, delivered fully online, and was an international study. They recommended not including the terms randomised controlled trials in the flyer. After numerous iterations of the flyer which went back and forth between the research team and the PPI group, we arrived at the final flyer.
>
> The HOMESIDE website was also a promotional product that we developed. We designed the site so there was a place to register your interest in study participation in addition to pages that provided updates on study progress, announcements of when milestones were achieved, and any media engagement piece. Past podcasts and recordings of webinars were also stored there and made available to the public.

Other promotional products include videos that can be posted to YouTube or Facebook or other social media. Again, it is vital to consider the content, length, and engagement of these videos, as its well understood that you have to catch the interest of your viewer within the first few seconds, otherwise they move on to something else. It is also recognised that ideally videos should be somewhere between 15 and 30 seconds. As with the flyer, make sure you test out the video, especially if you have access to a PPI committee whose members can provide invaluable feedback and might help shape the script. Market research tells us that it is good to utilise the same "advertisement" many times before considering changing to something new and fresh to keep people engaged. In our HOMESIDE study, we regularly revised our recruitment videos, introducing new images, trying out new styles of framing the research, and regularly consulting with our PPI committee to check our messaging was consistent with the project intentions but was also engaging and simple enough for the lay person to understand.

Promoting the Study

Once the promotional materials are ready for launching, the research team should consider what strategy will increase the visibility and reach of the study. This component of the strategy must feed directly from your understanding your participants daily activities and the locations (physical and virtual) where they are likely to "stumble" across the promotional materials developed for your research project. It is helpful to understand what media/social media, community participation, databases, government and not-for-profit organisations, your target population, or their gate keepers may interact with.

> *Case Example of Study Promotion.* In our HOMESIDE study, we utilised a series of different avenues to promote the study of people living with dementia and their family carers. These included:
>
> - Appearing on national television
> - Talking about the project on commercial and non-commercial radio
> - Professionally recorded podcasts promoted through the university media office
> - Presenting at family carers groups
> - Presenting to different stakeholder groups
> - Webinars describing the study, which included guest appearances from our trial therapists and past study participants
> - Disseminating flyers to home care provider organisations identified through government websites
> - Posters on noticeboards of community centres, churches, and other venues where people living with dementia frequent
> - Flyers disseminated at Dementia Cafes
> - Posting recruitment videos to dementia Facebook groups and YouTube and disseminating the links to our networks
> - Writing articles and creating paid advertisements in dementia care magazines
> - Presenting at relevant trade conferences.
>
> What we noted in HOMESIDE is that strategies worked differently across the different countries. For example, in Australia, Facebook was the most successful way of reaching our potential participant pool, followed by

> recruiting through a dementia-specific database where people register their interest in participating in research (StepUp https://www.stepupfordementiaresearch.org.au), and targeted radio interviews. In Germany, the most successful strategy was the placing of an article about the project in a free pharmacy magazine. In the UK, the National Institute for Health Research Clinical Research Network made a significant number of direct referrals, and the UK team also recruited through the Join Dementia Research (https://www.joindementiaresearch.nihr.ac.uk/) which is a database that links people interested in research with research teams. Digital tools such as social media and websites have been shown to increase the trial reach to participants in most studies (Blatch-Jones et al., 2020). Recruitment in Norway was most effective through engaging in targeted networks, while in Poland, venues such as churches were highly successful alongside Facebook advertisements and webinars. This highlights the differences that context (in this case country) can have on recruitment trends.

Continuous monitoring of recruitment trends is also imperative to identify which methods generate the most numbers of enrolments. This will help guide where to invest your time and effort. Similarly, monitoring which months of the year generate peaks and troughs in recruitment rates can help with recruitment planning. For example, in Europe, it might be difficult to recruit during July or August when people may be taking vacations and are unable to commit to the tasks or demands involved in research. Conversely, in Australia, Christmas and January are the times when people have holidays and are less likely to participate. Monitoring the geographical locations of recruited participants and correlating these with the promotional activities used can help to identify whether some geographical locations are more responsive to some recruitment methods compared with others. For example, as highlighted in Fig. 6.1, the StepUp database used to recruit in the HOMESIDE Australian study was particularly effective method of recruitment in the state of New South Wales, whereas posting advertisements on Facebook generated more interest in Queensland and Victoria. One of the best ways to capture this information is to develop a recruitment spreadsheet that captures the name, address, and location/type of promotional activity where potential participants learned about the study.

In terms of monitoring recruitment, once anticipated periods of peaks and troughs in recruitment rate have been identified, it can be helpful to have a week-by-week or month-by-month target, which can serve as

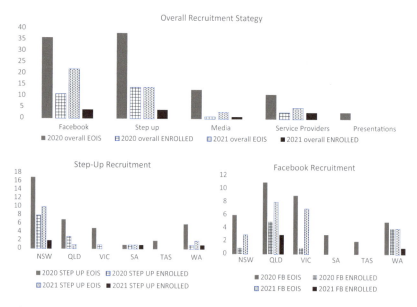

Fig. 6.1 Variability in effectiveness of recruitment strategies of the Australian cohort of the HOMESIDE trial

your barometer to assess how well your recruitment strategy is working. Without this active and continuous tracking of recruitment rates, it is very easy to fall behind in your targets.

For those research teams who are well resourced, you may want to consider planning a SWAT (Study Within A Trial) (Treweek et al., 2018) which I mentioned earlier in this chapter. This is a study that is nested within the larger clinical trial which intentionally compares the effectiveness of different recruitment strategies. To do this rigorously, the SWAT requires careful planning, a study protocol of its own, and non-biased randomisation processes. This will give you definitive evidence of the best recruitment strategies. At the time of writing this book, the HOMESIDE team had completed its SWAT on an evaluation of the effectiveness of their recruitment strategy (Baker et al. submitted). Alternatively, if resources (time and money) are more limited, the research team can undertake their own systematic review of how other researchers have promoted and recruited to their studies and draw on their work to determine what are the likely best strategies. Our HOMESIDE research team did exactly this and our findings informed our HOMESIDE recruitment strategy (Baker et al., 2021).

Price

I cannot emphasise enough, the need to allocate a generous budget for recruitment. Carefully considered investment in promotional materials (especially advertising) to expedite recruitment can be less expensive than with the cost associated with running a trial that is slow to recruit and at risk of being underpowered. It is not good use of finances (or time in an often time-bound study) to have paid members of a study team waiting for potential participants to enrol in the study. This is a waste of resources. So, it may be better to allocate funds towards an active recruitment strategy that has the research team proactively identifying and communicating with referral agencies or actively contacting potential participants themselves.

In developing the recruitment plan, one needs a clear idea of how much recruitment costs (particularly in staff time) to identify and discuss the project with a potential participant and convert this into a study enrolment. For example, in our MIDDEL study (Baker et al., 2020), we screened 666 people with dementia from which we enrolled 318 residents. In terms of resources, it took our recruiters an average of 1.67 (standard deviation = 1.14) phone call attempts to make the initial contact with participants' next of kin. Additionally, several follow-up emails and phone calls were needed to actually secure an enrolment, and it took an average 45.92 days (standard deviation = 46.79) before a formal consent was received. There was a significant amount of time and effort involved in (1) initiating contact, (2) keeping a log of what team member made the contact and when, and (3) scheduling follow-up phone calls (when needed). Such logs are critical in the recruitment monitoring to reduce the risk of losing eligible participants.

When planning the recruitment strategy and investing in promotional materials and fee-paying places to promote the study, it will be important to weigh up the costs of advertising with the conversion to a study enrolment—that is, what does it cost in promotional activities to recruit a participant. Huynh et al. (2014) undertook a systematic review of the cost-effectiveness of recruitment approaches undertaken in 10 randomised studies that compared recruitment strategies, including monetary incentives (cash or prize), direct contact (letters or telephone call), and medical referral strategies. Their study found that allocating additional resources to recruit participants using monetary incentives or directly contacting potential participants yielded between 4 and 23% additional participants compared to using neither strategy. Monetary incentives which ranged from US$1 to $200 cash, found that it cost between $3.47 to $57.69 per randomised participant. Direct contact via letter or phone call invitation was more economical and ranged from $0.93c (letters) to $15.30 (telephone calls). They found that the web-based advertisement generated the lowest cost per participant recruited ($18.56 per patient), whereas non-web-based adverts were significantly more expensive ($514.85 per patient).

Working with Industry Partners

Partner organisations are key gatekeepers that can block or advance your recruitment strategy. They may play a key role in referrals and/or screening. However, they can be a barrier if they have reservations about the study. Reservations may include concern: (1) for the degree of burden participants may experience, (2) for the health and wellbeing of the participants, (3) about the safety and potential harmful effects of the intervention, and (4) aspects of the study design particularly randomisation (Dunleavy et al., 2018). When working with partners, researchers may also experience that staff do not devote the required time to recruit to the project, or staff are unavailable because of vacation or changing work shifts, or staff turnover. These were certainly barriers we faced in our MIDDEL clinical trial in residential aged care homes (Baker et al., 2020).

Despite these challenges, there are simple practices that you can implement that increase the chances that partners will advance not limit your recruitment strategy. My first recommendation is to start with securing buy-in from an organisation's management team such as the general manager, medical director, or school principal. When approaching them, consider opening the communication with a statement about what problem their consumers/patients might have, and how you have a potential solution. In our MIDDEL study, we developed an information package that included (1) a statement about the need for addressing the high incidence of depression in residential aged care homes, (2) a statement about how we had the solution to this and what that solution was, (3) a statement about what partnering with us could mean for their organisation, and (4) what partnership would look like. Our statements included highlighting that partnership would include us providing them with AUS$10,000 of free music interventions over 6 months per care home, which would lead to wellbeing outcomes for their residents and healthcare staff, publicity opportunities, and being part of a large potentially policy-changing trial. We approached and signed up four leading aged care providers who partnered with us to implement the study across 40 residential aged care homes.

Once you have secured a partner, the relationship does not end there. To optimise the partnership, it is important that staff in the partner organisation fully understands the aims and benefits of the research, what is involved and what their responsibilities are, and how the research team and the partner organisation can work together to identify and recruit study participants. To achieve this, educating the partner organisation through site visits and provision of staff education sessions on the project will help to deepen their understanding of the project. Allow plenty of time for them to ask questions, and opportunities to reassure them of any concerns they might have about the study. My experience has been that you often can identify a "champion" among the staff, a person who truly recognises the value of the project and is willing to support your efforts. These champions are like nuggets of gold that you should nurture all the way throughout the trial (Baker et al., 2020).

Repeated communication is needed to ensure partner motivation and energy is sustained throughout the study. I have utilised several strategies to achieve this. Firstly, in our MIDDEL study in residential aged care homes (Baker et al., 2020), we funded an additional care home staff member to be on site on the days we were screening/assessing potential participants to expedite the recruitment process. We also delivered gourmet hampers of chocolates and fruit at random times to show our ongoing recognition of partner contributions to the project.

Involvement of Public and Patients in Recruitment

The value of involving the PPI committee in recruitment can extend beyond the design of promotional materials. Crocker et al. (2015) conducted a systematic review and meta-analysis on the impact of PPI on study enrolment and found that on average, having people with lived experience actively recruiting participants, significantly increased the chances of a person enrolling in a clinical trial. This is because people with lived experience are best placed to understand how to reach the target population. Crocker et al. (2015) also found that PPI in recruitment serves to overcome barriers of stigma and mistrust.

Strategies to Improve Conversion Rates

While raising awareness of the research to the potential pool of participants and attracting their interest is perhaps the most essential component of recruitment, there is little point in having high interest if only a small percentage of them convert to a study enrolment. In many of my studies, I have experienced high numbers of eligible participants, but for various reasons, converting them into an actual enrolment was challenging, time-consuming, and at times frustrating. After reviewing the literature and based on my own experiences, there seems to be a few key strategies that increase the chances of a conversion, notwithstanding unavoidable contextual factors. The strategies are harnessing trust, supporting participants during the decision-making process, minimising burden of participation, and demonstrating respect and value for their contribution (Natale et al., 2021).

Harness Trust

As highlighted earlier, scepticism, fear, and mistrust are barriers to study enrolment, so researchers need to consider strategies for building trust with potential participants. A good starting point is to work closely with partner organisations and referring clinicians, because participants are more likely to "trust" participation recommendations that come from them, than direct invitations from the research team (Natale et al., 2021). The potential participants' own treatment teams can be a valuable resource because they can discuss the value of the trial with them and help them to weigh up the benefits against the burden and potential risks.

Supporting Decision Making

Before feeling comfortable to make the decision to enrol, participants need to feel well informed about the aims of the study, what the potential benefits are for participation, and the time commitment involved (Natale et al., 2021). The recruitment team can implement several strategies to ensure this is the case. First and foremost, optimise the trial information sheet by using plain language with accessible wording, visual aids such as icons or pictures, contrasting colours where possible, and larger font sizes that make reading easier (Liu et al., 2018) (as described earlier).

When you have a large percentage of potential participants with a first language that differs to that of the larger community, try to allocate some of the budget to have the trial information sheet translated into the most common languages (Masood et al., 2019). Another strategy is to engage translator, or better still, have members of the research team that are bilingual (Masood et al., 2019). A study that we have in planning at present is an extension of the MATCH study, which will take our eHealth application and assess, modify, and validate its effectiveness with people from different cultural backgrounds to ensure generalisability of the application. This idea emerged from our HOMESIDE team in Norway where we noted that there was only a small number of participants who were not native-born Norwegians, enrolled in the study. We want to address the under-representation and are planning to intentionally employ participants from targeted cultural groups to join the research team as recruiters. Based on the literature, we envisage that this will allow our potential participants to feel more comfortable with the study team and more likely to enrol.

Participating in research is a big decision that requires careful consideration. Researchers can assist people in making the decision by giving them plenty of time to make the decision and offering to answer questions. Be prepared to answer the same question over and over, if that is what is needed for them to arrive at a decision.

Minimise Burden of Participation

Every participant's personal, health, and family context is different, so be aware of their circumstances and context and consider how you might be able to adapt materials or processes to reduce burden and accommodate contextual factors (Natale et al., 2021). The research team can adopt several approaches to achieve this. Firstly, consider the participants other commitments and try to accommodate that into your schedule rather than the reverse. For example, for those that are working during business hours, schedule appointments after hours. If they are parents of young children, schedule appointments during school hours. Be conscious of their need to take vacations, attend family or religious events, and accommodate these into the research schedule accordingly. Where remote participation is possible, offer this as an alternative as it can minimise the burden associated with travel. If possible, offer financial reimbursement for costs incurred in relation to participation. This could include taxi fares, parking fees, or meals. These considerations may help allay any concerns they may have about their willingness and capacity to commit to the project.

Offering Appropriate Incentives

It is becoming much more common now for participants to receive incentives for their participation that are above and beyond the potential health benefits of the intervention received. Incentives can take the form of cash payments, vouchers to clubs or restaurants, store gift cards, or movie tickets. Some studies offer participants the possibility of winning something of value like an iPad, a weekend away, or a meal at a fancy restaurant. When planning what type of incentive and what amounts to offer, one needs to make sure that the financial gain does not become the reason for choosing to enrol. We want participants to enrol in the research because they feel they could benefit from the research participation and that they want to contribute to the knowledge about interventions that support better health and wellbeing. If the financial gain is too large, we risk biasing our sample. At the same time, financial incentives should be sufficiently matched to the amount of effort, involvement, and potential vulnerability that the person may be subjected to. For example, studies requiring two hours per week of participation over four months should receive a higher financial incentive than those that participate for two hours per week for four weeks.

Working with Your Recruitment Team

As someone who has been a recruiter and been recruited to trials, I have come to recognise that the way people communicate with potential participants can be the make or break of converting an expression of interest to participate into a study enrolment. Feedback from participants has been that who, how, and when a recruiter approaches them is critical in their decision to go ahead with participation. When the person you are recruiting is unknown to the recruiter, communication style is essential in building confidence and trust. Brown et al. (2014) suggest that recruiters who are warm, friendly, and interested in their participants' wellbeing are more likely to convert a potential participant into an enrolment. Raven-Gregg et al. (2021) and Baker et al. (2020) suggest that a positive, empathic approach combined with the recruiter taking time to thoroughly explain the need for research will increase the chances of study enrolment. It is also important when engaging with potential participants, to practise therapeutic listening and allow them to share stories of strengths and concerns. This can be time-consuming but ultimately is more likely to lead to a study enrolment (Baker et al., 2020).

A recruitment script that has been tested to ensure messaging in ordered correctly, presented sensitively, and is used consistently may also increase the chances of recruitment success (Baker et al., 2020). In our residential aged care home trial, we were required to obtain consent from next of kin because the majority of participants with dementia were unable to provide informed consent to participate. Our data indicated that the order of study information provided was correlated with a willingness to consent to study participation. For example, we discovered early on in our recruitment phase that explaining the need to collect data on medication use (an obviously sensitive topic) should be presented very late in the discussion, when there was a clear sense that the next of kin were on board with study participation. Similarly, to avoid being shut down early in the communication, we needed to articulate early that even people who are in the later stages of dementia are still able to participate in music and that special musical skills are not required for participation. Further, our reflections were that we needed to come across as sounding cheerful, professional, and knowledgeable but not overly formal. We experimented with the script and found that the most effective order was to state:

1. Your discipline (in my case music therapy)
2. You are a researcher from The University of X
3. Your research team has a collaboration with X organisation and
4. You are wanting to discuss the participation of X (name of resident) in the study of….

I cannot stress enough how important the initial conversations are. In training your research team, it is important to spend time role playing and testing out the scripts.

Barriers to Participant Retention and Follow-Up

Now you have your participant in the study, the next challenge is to keep them in the study. Attrition is a reality of every trial and some attrition is unavoidable. Many trials may lose participants due to a change in health status pointing to a change in their eligibility, or because of declining health that precludes participation, or worse, death (Forsat et al., 2020; Song et al., 2021). In our HOMESIDE trial based in residential aged care, we lost 118 of our 318 participants to death (37%) (many of whom died because of COVID-19). However, some participant attrition can be minimised with careful planning.

Attrition can occur when participants lose engagement with the project (Forsat et al., 2020; Song et al., 2021). What seemed like an altruistic and noble thing to do in the first instance became somewhat of a hassle, especially once the novelty of participation had worn off. Attrition may also occur for contextual reasons such as having competing family obligations, work commitments, challenges in accessing transportation to study site, or they simply just forget about the study because they become caught up in their everyday lives (Bonevski et al., 2014; Forsat et al., 2020; Song et al., 2021). Researchers need to be aware that while our participants are essential to meeting the study aims, participation may not be a priority for our participants. An awareness and respect for that is necessary at all times.

Adverse events or negative intervention effects are additional reasons why participants may withdraw. Serious adverse events may be related to the intervention under investigation (e.g. outburst of anger or frustration that requires additional interventions, emotional breakdown requiring referrals to counselling) or totally unrelated (e.g. an unplanned emergency visit to hospital). Such events may lead to the study team withdrawing the participant. Non-serious adverse effects are those that may be anticipated due to the nature of the intervention, which cause feelings of vulnerability, distress, or feeling overwhelmed. For example, psychological distress may arise when asking personal questions as part of the standardised data collection processes. In my own experience, some questions on depression scales may occasionally distress participants, especially (but not exclusively) people with cognitive impairment who may not be able to fully appreciate or comprehend why the questions are being posed. Questions about suicide (framed as "taking your own life") have been distressing and offensive for some participants, causing a withdrawal from study participation.

Factors to Increase Retention

While researchers may have no capacity to impact the health status of participants or their experience of adverse events, they can play an important role in maintaining a participants' engagement and commitment to the project. Perhaps the most effective strategy is for the study team to regularly communicate with participants (Forsat et al., 2020). Communication might take the form of a person-centred approach such as a phone call to check in on them. Our experiences are that for many people with chronic health conditions, having a person they can spend some minutes with talking about their health problems can be helpful in keeping them engaged in the study. These moments of contact provide a simple and cost-effective opportunity for the research team to express their appreciation of their contribution, thereby helping to maintain the participants' commitment to sustained engagement in the project.

Communication may also take the form of a more formal approach such as sending out a regular newsletter which offers participants an update on the progress of the study. Such actions have also been shown to sustain engagement in the study (Bonevski et al., 2014). More recently, social media has been used to communicate study updates and help participants feel connected to the project. These might include Twitter or Facebook posts, and/or a central website where study information and updates can be viewed by participants. All these initiatives are effective in lowering attrition.

Financial incentives are a means to sustain participant engagement. I have found it helpful to have a staggered approach to payments when participation occurs over a longer period. For example, in our MATCH project which is developing a music-based mobile application for managing agitation in people living with dementia, we engaged people with lived experience to complete a short survey, and later, in participate in two to three 2-hour workshops spread across several months. To increase engagement, we staggered the financial incentives across different phases of the study period. Following completion of the survey, participants entered into a draw to win an iPad. And following each workshop, people were paid for their participation.

Motivating the Recruitment Team

Tracking and celebrating reaching recruitment milestones will help sustain team motivation as they can see their efforts moving them ever closer towards the end goal. This should be the aim of every research leader. However, the reality may be quite different. I have encountered that recruitment can be very stressful for the research team, especially when recruitment rate is slow or at worst stagnant, and the trial appears to be falling behind schedule. Stress is exacerbated when one study site or one single recruiter has recruited larger numbers of participants compared with the others. Some authors believe that instilling a healthy sense of competition between sites or recruiters can help sustain motivation during the recruitment phase of the trial (Forsat et al., 2020; Liu et al., 2018), however my experience is counter to that. Motivation is sustained when the team meet regularly to share ideas, frustrations, and create new recruitment strategies together. This instils more team ownership of the process and views the study tasks as a shared responsibility. In turn, this builds a sense of "we-ness" rather than a "me-ness" or "other-ness" which will help the team members move through the low points in the recruitment period.

Conclusion

Recruitment is challenging for every research project, and the larger the trial, the more challenging it becomes. However, with the right strategies and monitoring in place, recruitment targets can be met. It is imperative that the team expect peaks and troughs otherwise they can become despondent when recruitment is slow. Noticing the trends of when the peaks occur can allow the team to strategise how to maximise recruitment during those peak periods.

References

Ahmed, A., Vandrevala, T., Hendy, J., Kelly, C., & Ala, A. (2019). An examination of how to engage migrants in the research process: Building trust through an "insider" perspective. *Ethnicity & Health*. https://doi.org/10.1080/13557858.2019.1685651

Altman, D. G. (1994). The scandal of poor medical research. *British Medical Journal, 308*(6924), 283–284.

Baker, F. (2001). The effects of live, taped and no music on people experiencing posttraumatic amnesia. *Journal of Music Therapy, 38*(3), 170–192.

Baker, F. (2011). Facilitating neurological reorganization through music therapy: A case example of modified melodic intonation therapy in the treatment of a person with aphasia. In A. Meadows (Ed.), *Developments in music therapy practice: Case perspectives* (pp. 281–297). Phoenixville.

Baker, F. A., Bloska, J., Stensæth, K., Wosch, T., Bukowska, A., Braat, S., Sousa, T., Tamplin, J., Clark, I. N., Lee, Y.-E. C., Clarke, P., Lautenschlager, N., & Odell-Miller, H. (2019). HOMESIDE: A home-based family caregiver-delivered music intervention for people living with dementia: Protocol of a randomised controlled trial. *British Medical Journal Open.* https://doi.org/10.1136/bmjopen-2019-031332

Baker, F.A., Lee, Y.-E. C., Sousa, T. V., Stretton-Smith, P. A., Tamplin, J., Sveinsdottir, V., Geretsegger, M., Wake, J. D., Assmus, J., Christian Gold, C. (2022). Clinical effectiveness of Music Interventions for Dementia and Depression in Elderly care (MIDDEL) in the Australian cohort: Pragmatic cluster-randomised controlled trial. *The Lancet Healthy Longevity, 3*(3), e153–e165.

Baker, F. A., Pool, J., Johansson, K., Wosch, T., Bukowska, A. A., Kulis, A., Blauth, L., Stensæth, K., Clark, I. N., & Odell-Miller, H. (2021). Strategies for recruiting people with dementia to music therapy studies: Systematic review. *Journal of Music Therapy.* https://doi.org/10.1093/jmt/thab010

Baker, F. A., Stretton-Smith, P., Sousa, T. A., Clark, I., Cotton, A., Gold, C., & Lee, Y.-E. C. (2020). Process and resource assessment in trials undertaken in residential care homes: Experiences from the Australian MIDDEL research team. *Contemporary Clinical Trials Communication.* https://doi.org/10.1016/j.conctc.2020.100675

Baker, F. A., Tamplin, J., Rickard, N., Ponsford, J., New, P., & Lee, Y.-E. C. (2019). A therapeutic songwriting intervention to promote reconstruction of self-concept and enhance wellbeing following brain and spinal cord injury: Pilot randomised controlled trial. *Clinical Rehabilitation.* https://doi.org/10.1177/0123456789123456. First Published 22 February 2019.

Blatch-Jones, A., Nuttall, J., Bull, A., Worswick, L., Mullee, M., Peveler, R., Falk, S., Tape, N., Hinks, J., Lane, A. J., Wyatt, J. C., & Griffiths, G. (2020). Using digital tools in the recruitment and retention in randomised controlled trials: Survey of UK Clinical Trial Units and a qualitative study. *Trials, 21*(1). https://doi.org/10.1186/s13063-020-04234-0

Bonevski, B., Randell, M., Paul, C., Chapman, K., Twyman, L., Bryant, J., Brozek, I., & Hughes, C. (2014). Reaching the hard-to-reach: A systematic review of strategies for improving health and medical research with socially disadvantaged groups. *BMC Medical Research Methodology, 14.* https://doi.org/10.1186/1471-2288-14-42

Brown, G., Marshall, M., Bower, P., Woodham, A., & Waheed, W. (2014). Barriers to recruiting ethnic minorities to mental health research: A systematic review. *International Journal of Methods in Psychiatric Research, 23*(1), 36–48. https://doi.org/10.1002/mpr.1434

Chalmers, I., & Glasziou, P. (2009). Avoidable waste in the production and reporting of research evidence. *Obstetrics and Gynaecology, 114*, 1341–1345. https://doi.org/10.1097/AOG.0b013e3181c3020d

Cook, C., & Sheets, C. (2011). Clinical equipoise and personal equipoise: Two necessary ingredients for reducing bias in manual therapy trials. *Journal of Manual and Manipulative Therapy, 1*, 55.

Crocker, J., Hughes-Morley, A., Petit-Zeman, S., & Rees, S. (2015). Assessing the impact of patient and public involvement on recruitment and retention in clinical trials: A systematic review. *Trials, 16*(Suppl 2). https://doi.org/10.1186/1745-6215-16-S2-O91

Dunleavy, L., Walshe, C., Oriani, A., & Preston, N. (2018). Using the "Social Marketing Mix Framework" to explore recruitment barriers and facilitators in palliative care randomised controlled trials? A narrative synthesis review. *Palliative Medicine, 32*(5), 990–1009.

Forsat, N. D., Palmowski, A., Palmowski, Y., Boers, M., & Buttgereit, F. (2020). Recruitment and retention of older people in clinical research: A systematic literature review. *Journal of the American Geriatrics Society, 68*(12), 2955–2963. https://doi.org/10.1111/jgs.16875

Gardner, H. (2018). *Making clinical trials more efficient: Consolidating, communicating and improving knowledge of participant recruitment interventions.* PhD Thesis. University of Aberdeen.

Gold, C., Eickholt, J., Assmus, J., Stige, B., Wake, J. D., Baker, F. A., Tamplin, J., Clark, I., Lee, Y.-E., Jacobsen, S. J., Ridder, H. M. O., Kreutz, G., Muthesius, D., Wosch, T., Ceccato, E., Raglio, A., Ruggeri, M., Vink, A., Zuidema, S., ... Geretsegger, M. (2019). Music Interventions for Dementia and Depression in ELderly care (MIDDEL): Protocol and statistical analysis plan for a multinational cluster-randomised trial. *British Medical Journal Open, 9*(3). https://doi.org/10.1136/bmjopen-2018-023436

Huynh, L., Johns, B., Liu, S.-H., Vedula, S. S., Li, T., & Puhan, M. A. (2014). Cost-effectiveness of health research study participant recruitment strategies: A systematic review. *Clinical Trials, 11*(5), 576–583. https://doi.org/10.1177/1740774514540371

LeBlanc, T. W., Lodato, J. E., Currow, D. C., & Abernethy, A. P. (2013). Overcoming recruitment challenges in palliative care clinical trials. *Journal of Oncology Practice, 9*, 277–282.

Lee, Y. E., Sousa, T. V., Stretton-Smith, P. A., Gold, C., Geretsegger, M., & Baker, F. A. (2022). Profile of residents living in residential aged care with dementia and depression: Data from the MIDDEL cluster-randomised controlled trial. *Australasian Journal of Ageing*. https://doi.org/10.1111/ajag.13104

Lidz, C. W., & Appelbaum, P. S. (2002). The therapeutic misconception: Problems and solutions. *Medical Care, 40*(9), V55–V63.
Liu, Y., Pencheon, E., Hunter, R. M., Moncrieff, J., & Freemantle, N. (2018). Recruitment and retention strategies in mental health trials—A systematic review. *PLoS ONE, 13*(8), 1–17. https://doi.org/10.1371/journal.pone.0203127
Masood, Y., Bower, P., Waheed, M. W., Brown, G., & Waheed, W. (2019). Synthesis of researcher reported strategies to recruit adults of ethnic minorities to clinical trials in the United Kingdom: A systematic review. *Contemporary Clinical Trials, 78*, 1–10. https://doi.org/10.1016/j.cct.2019.01.004
McDonald, M., Townsend, A., Cox, S. M., Paterson, N. D., & Lafreniere, D. (2008). Trust in health research relationships: Accounts of human subjects. *Journal of Empirical Research on Human Research Ethics, 3*(4), 35–47.
Naidoo, N., Nguyen, V. T., Ravaud, P., Young, B., Amiel, P., Schante, D., Clarke, M., & Boutron, I. (2020). The research burden of randomized controlled trial participation: A systematic thematic synthesis of qualitative evidence. *BMC Medicine, 18*(1). https://doi.org/10.1186/s12916-019-1476-5
Natale, P., Saglimbene, V., Ruospo, M., Gonzalez, A. M., Strippoli, G. F., Scholes-Robertson, N., Guha, C., Craig, J. C., Teixeira-Pinto, A., Snelling, T., & Tong, A. (2021). Transparency, trust and minimizing burden to increase recruitment and retention in trials: A systematic review. *Journal of Clinical Epidemiology, 134*, 35. https://doi.org/10.1016/j.jclinepi.2021.01.014
National Institute of Health (NIH). (2004). Guidelines on the inclusion of women and minorities as subjects in clinical research. *NIH Guide, 23*, 2–3.
Nichols, L., Martindale-Adams, J., Burns, R., Coon, D., Ory, M., Mahoney, D., Tarlow, B., Burgio, L., Gallagher-Thompson, D., Guy, D., Arguelles, T., & Winter, L. (2004). Social marketing as a framework for recruitment: Illustrations from the REACH study. *Journal of Aging Health, 16*, 157S–176S.
Raven-Gregg, T., Wood, F., & Shepherd, V. (2021). Effectiveness of participant recruitment strategies for critical care trials: A systematic review and narrative synthesis. *Clinical Trials, 18*(4), 436–448.
Song, L., Qan'ir, Y., Guan, T., Guo, P., Xu, S., Jung, A., Idiagbonya, E., Song, F., & Kent, E. E. (2021). The challenges of enrolment and retention: A systematic review of psychosocial behavioral interventions for patients with cancer and their family caregivers. *Journal of Pain and Symptom Management.* https://doi.org/10.1016/j.jpainsymman.2021.04.019
Teemil, Z. (2019). *An investigation of how healthcare organisations use social media as marketing tools in the UK: The case of private and social care organisations.* https://search.ebscohost.com/login.aspx?direct=true&AuthType=sso&db=edsble&AN=edsble.794455&site=eds-live&scope=site. Accessed 8 August 2021.

Treweek, S., Pitkethly, M., Cook, J., Fraser, C., Mitchell, E., Sullivan, R., Jackson, C., Taskila, T. K., & Gardner, H. (2018). Strategies to improve recruitment to randomised trials. *Cochrane Database Systematic Review*, 2:MR000013. https://doi.org/10.1002/14651858.MR000013.pub6

UyBico, S. J., Pavel, S., & Gross, C. P. (2007). Recruiting vulnerable populations into research: A systematic review of recruitment interventions. *Journal of General Internal Medicine, 22*(6), 852. https://doi.org/10.1007/s11606-007-0126-3

CHAPTER 7

Quality Data Is Power: Data Management and Monitoring

THE NEED FOR GOOD DATA MANAGEMENT AND MONITORING

A successful trial, irrespective of whether the hypotheses are supported or rejected, is one where the trial has been implemented according to the protocol, the data collected is precise and valid, the statistical analyses selected are appropriate, and the results accurately interpreted for clinical application. After all, research conclusions are only as good as the data upon which they were based (Zozus et al., 2019).

Good data management and monitoring is also needed for compliance with ethical regulations. The Declaration of Helsinki (World Medical Association, 2018) states that all trials adhere to good clinical practice guidelines (ICH, 2021), which includes monitoring the trial to ensure it is compliant with international regulations, standards, and guidelines. The monitoring should involve rigorous reviews of data to ensure all procedures are implemented consistently and safely throughout the trial. A rigorous data management plan (DMP, now usually a requirement for ethical approvals) will make preparing for audits and reporting simpler and more streamlined. In this chapter, the focus is on the development of the DMP, the collection of data, the setting up of data collection processes to safeguard quality data collection, and descriptions of how to monitor the data over the duration of the trial.

Defining Quality Data

Quality data has been broadly defined as "fitness for use"—in other words, the data is able to be analysed so that the research hypotheses posed can be tested and inferences made by the results derived from the analyses (Zozus et al., 2019). There is a consensus that quality data (or a data set) contains data that is reliable and valid. This means the data needs to be accurate (the value recorded is the true value of what is being measured), complete (missing data is minimal), and collected in a way that promotes trustworthiness (for example, assessors are masked to allocation). Throughout the trial, multiple people may be involved in collecting, handling, and processing data, all of whom can influence the quality of the data during any one or all of these steps. Zozus et al. (2019) state that the gold standard in planning for data management and monitoring is to set up processes that aim to prevent errors in data, rather than relying on an "after-the-fact checking process to find and fix errors". Here, a plan for prevention rather than treatment of arriving at a quality data set is warranted.

In the case of observing and measuring data, it is important that the processes are set up to minimise the chances of incorrect or biased measurements. Where appropriate, this can be achieved by multiple testing or measuring the same construct using two different questions within a questionnaire. Data quality is also at risk from lack of consistency between multiple assessors, particularly if data is based on potentially subjective observation of behaviour as is often the case in trials involving the creative arts therapies. Extensive assessor training and an assessment of interrater reliability will be needed to ensure accurate data is collected. In our MIDDEL project (Baker et al., 2022), we created a series of assessor training tools including a detailed manual and conducted several interrater reliability tests throughout the trial to ensure consistency between assessors.

Recording data in a clear and consistent manner is also important for ensuring data quality. Processes should be put in place so that (1) the source of data is always clearly identified, (2) the source should be protected so it cannot be altered, lost, or destroyed, and (3) good documentation practices are adopted including legibility of the data, not obscuring the original value when a change is made, and documentation of who made any change (Zozus et al., 2019).

Levels of Data Monitoring

There are four main levels of data monitoring within a trial, each serving their own purpose during trial implementation: (1) high level monitoring at governance level, (2) central monitoring at operational level, (3) statistical level monitoring, and (4) site specific monitoring. *High-level monitoring* refers to the monitoring of data at the pooled data level from various governance committees (see Chapter 3 for extensive descriptions of the committees' roles and responsibilities). The Trial Steering Committee uses available data to review the progress of all important aspects of the trial including timelines, deliverables, completeness of data sets, recruitment, and participant flow through the study, budgets, and other aspects of trial delivery. From the review, they provide high-level advice on trial progress which helps the Trial Management Group make strategic decisions about executing any actions or adaptations needed to progress the trial. Similarly, high-level monitoring is performed by the Data Safety Monitoring Board who intermittently carefully review the available data to identify any safety concerns highlighted via documented adverse events, unexpected and serious adverse events, and mortality. They may also review the integrity and rigor of the trial implementation processes. They can offer feedback to the Trial Management Group about any concerns they may have to participant safety, the quality (accuracy, completeness, integrity) of the data collected, and make recommendations for modifications or for trial continuation or discontinuation as they see necessary (see Chapter 3).

While some data collection can be automated, humans collect and record most of the data in creative arts therapies trials. Consequently, when humans are required to observe participants engaging in performing arts or read aloud the test questions to participants, human error and variability are likely. Regular *central level monitoring*—monitoring performed by the research team who operationalise a trial—is needed to identify and rectify errors. Here, data are reviewed firstly by the data manager, and then when issues are found, additional information is sought by members of the team to reconcile inconsistencies or obvious errors, and to check whether missing data is actually missing as opposed to not yet having been entered into the database. When monitoring participant flow through the study and its associated data, the review may involve checking that: (1) the data collection forms have been completed correctly (signed, dated), (2) the database entries have been reviewed and verified, (3) the success of intervention adherence is documented, and (4) the intervention and assessor fidelity checks have been implemented and documented. Regular central level monitoring can work as a preventative tool, signalling frequently to the research team, the need for "good" data collection, handling, and processing. Importantly, central level monitoring can extend beyond participant flow and data tracking. It may focus on the success of assessor masking, severity and number of protocol violations, resource use (for budget strategy), staff training and supervision, staff holiday leave, governance reporting, and timelines and deliverables.

The central monitoring is usually planned to take place at pre-specified timepoints. The scope and complexity of the trial will dictate how often reviews need to take place. In the case of our HOMESIDE trial (Baker, Bloska, et al., 2019), we planned monthly monitoring of the recruitment data because we needed frequent overviews of how each country was performing. However, quarterly monitoring reviews for the remainder of the data was considered sufficient for tracking participant flow. Conversely, in the MIDDEL trial, recruitment occurred in waves (intensively every three to four months) so was not tracked regularly but sporadically. Further, due to the intensive and longitudinal nature of the intervention (up to four sessions per week over 3 months and two sessions per week over the subsequent 3 months), monthly reviews were vital to ensure the team were across any issues as they arose (Baker et al., 2022).

Monitoring Informed Consent—A Case Example. Molloy and Henley's (2016) practical guide for developing a DMP highlights the importance of monitoring informed consent procedures. These processes can be divided into two main components: the *development* of participant information sheets and consent forms, and the *completion* of the consent form. For the development of forms, monitoring processes need to be established to check that each participant has signed the correct version approved by ethics and that any language translations and back translations have been performed for those consent forms translated into different languages. In other words, has the right form been signed? This may seem like an unnecessary process as one might assume that members of the research team are providing the correct consent form for signing. However, this assumption was tested in one of my own studies—the Singing My Story (Baker, Tamplin, Rickard, et al., 2019) project. During the trial, a series of amendments had been submitted for ethical approval, some resulting in modifications to the consent forms. For example, any time a new researcher was added to the team, we needed to add their name to the consent form and therefore submit an ethics amendment with the revised form. At one point during the trial, our team was randomly selected for audit by the ethics committee. Following the review, the auditors discovered that several consent forms were signed using superseded forms. Somehow there was a breakdown in our organisational and communication processes because one staff member, who was involved in recruitment, had not been provided with an updated version. Once identified, we were able to correct the error for the remainder of the trial. If we had a better monitoring and self-audit process in place, we may have identified this error earlier rather than having it identified by an independent auditor.

In addition to monitoring the completion of the correct consent form, the research team need to also monitor whether the form has been fully completed. The team should also check that the form has the participant study number clearly documented, the appropriate people have signed the form (participant and/or legal guardian), and the date on the form is the same as the date of enrolment. Checks must also be put in place to ensure that the participant providing consent has capacity to consent (cognitively able to at time consent was sought). In our MIDDEL study, we rarely had participants who had capacity to provide consent. The consent process was complex because at times there were two different legal guardians—one for financial issues, and a separate person for consent to medical care. We also had two separate consent forms to sign. The first was a form to participate in the study, and the second form was a standardised form by the Department of Human Services. A signature on the latter form was needed for the study team to access participant medical care and medication use from federally managed Medicare Database. During our monitoring and checking processes, we found at times that consent forms had been signed by the financial rather than medical guardian. Further, at times, only one form was returned to the study team. Regular checking of the consenting process enabled the team to identify when incorrect or incomplete consent forms were returned so these could be followed up.

The third layer of monitoring is at the *statistical level*. Here, data is intermittently reviewed by the data manager and biostatistical team, to ensure the data is complete, plausible, reliable, and valid. By reviewing entered scores across a data set, the team can identify invalid, unexpected, or abnormal values which may signal human error. For example, possible participant scores on a single questionnaire item or the total score of a questionnaire may range from zero (minimum score) to 7 (maximum score). The statistical level review will highlight whether there are any scores are outside that range indicating the entry is invalid and in need of checking. Statistical reviews are also used to identify whether any entered values are rounded up or down, and whether there are any unusual frequency distributions (mean, variance, skewness). For multisite or international trials where on-site monitoring is not feasible, statistical monitoring through comparison of data between sites may be useful in highlighting issues related to a single site.

On-site monitoring is whereby processes and procedures are checked at the study sites where the study implementation is taking place. In many cases, data collected offsite (i.e. not at the university where the study team is located) will need to be stored at the site where it is collected—for example in a hospital. It is important that the research teams are confident that data and intervention implementation are being collected, delivered, and documented according to the study protocol and ethical guidelines. To be certain, at predefined intervals, a member of the research team should visit the site to cross-check that what has been recorded in the study's database, matches what is recorded at the data collection site, as well as matching the protocol, manual of operational procedures, and principles of good clinical practice.

The Data Management Plan (DMP)

The data management plan (DMP) is a document that describes the data the trial will generate during the trial implementation phase, and how the research team will manage, describe, and store the data, and the mechanisms and processes that will be adopted at the end of the project to share and preserve the data. The DMP should reliably collect and manage data that will enable the planned statistical analysis to be conducted and to safeguard compliance with the study protocol. The DMP protocol must also be compliant with ethical regulations including data collection, storage, protection, retention, and reporting of data. The DMP document may be a stand-alone document but is often included as a subsection within the Manual of Operational Procedures (MOP) (Chapter 2).

The content of the DMP will vary depending upon the complexity of the trial design and the number of sites where data is collected. Commonly included items in the plan are listed in Table 7.1. Each one of these components will be described in detail later in the chapter.

Table 7.1 Contents of a Data Management Plan

DMP section	Item description
Project Description	Brief description of aims, hypotheses, study design, participants, and study sites of the trial
Systems for Data Collection and Management	Description of systems for managing data including electronic database, and who will be responsible for building and managing it
Type of Data and Measures	Outlines the type of data being captured in the trial, for example standardised tools, biomarkers, brain imaging data, video, and interviews. For the creative arts therapies, this might also include artistic outputs such as artwork, song recordings, or performances (dance, drama, music),
Data Collection Method	Processes involved in collecting data including who collects the data, when, and in what format
Data Entry	Processes for entering data in the database
Data Security	
Data Cleaning and Quality Control	
Case Report Forms	
Data Access/Roles and Responsibilities	Research members who will have access to data, and what data each team member will access (e.g. assessors and those providing the creative arts therapy interventions may access different data)
Data Storage	How, where, and in what form (identifiable, re-identifiable, de-identified, etc.) data is stored
Confidentiality risks	Risks to breaches of confidentiality during data collection, data entry, and data storage that might occur
Study Participant Monitoring	Monitoring of participants through study period including: Screening/recruitment Randomisation/Blinding procedures Cessation of Intervention Withdrawals Tracking

(continued)

Table 7.1 (continued)

DMP section	Item description
Reporting	Processes for reporting data including: Safety, Adverse Events, Serious Adverse events Screening and Enrolment Data Quality and Completeness Progress and Final Reports Other reports as needed
Data Sharing	Descriptions whether de-identified data will be made available to others for reuse. Descriptions should include the format of data (pooled vs at individual participant level), and where and when that data will be made available

SYSTEMS FOR DATA COLLECTION AND MANAGEMENT

The novice or sole creative arts therapy researcher (as in a doctoral or postdoctoral researcher), they will mostly be leading small and contained clinical trials with modest sized participant samples and a limited amount of data. Managing data using simple tools such as Microsoft Excel spreadsheets is feasible in such contexts and can be easily imported into a statistical software program such as SPSS or R for analysis. However, with increasing complexity and the larger sample sizes of adequately powered clinical trials, creative arts therapy researchers may need to make use of more sophisticated data management systems and database tools. This will assist in systematically collecting, managing, and monitoring large amounts of data, and minimise the number of errors or missing data.

Electronic data capture (EDC) systems such as REDCap, Open Clinica, Castor, and Flex Databases (to name a few) are being increasingly adopted in large trials. These systems are designed to support the collection of data throughout the trial including the conduct, recording, evaluation, reporting, and archiving of the trial (ICH, 2021). Harris et al. (2009, p. 377) outlines the main features of EDC systems that support clinical trials:

1. collaborative access to data across academic departments and institutions thereby allowing multiple people to enter, access, monitor, and analyse data in a single secure place located in the cloud;

2. user authentication and role-based security so tracking of entries by staff member can occur;
3. intuitive electronic case report forms (CRFs) that prevent invalid values to be entered and reduced risk of missing data and ensure data is collected in the right order[1];
4. real-time data validation, integrity checks and other mechanisms for ensuring data quality (e.g. double-data entry options);
5. data attribution and audit capabilities to enable quick and easy identification of potentially inaccurate/missing data;
6. protocol document storage and sharing;
7. central data storage and backups;
8. data export functions for common statistical packages;
9. data import functions to facilitate bulk import of data from other systems.

Later in this chapter, I will describe the features of such databases and illustrate with screenshots how advantageous they are in monitoring the trial. It is important to note that these databases are not standardised or fixed but individually designed and constructed by the research team so as they meet the data management needs specific to that trial. Unlike other large digital health systems such as those implemented in the healthcare sector, an EDC in a trial is "self-contained, time-limited, and only accessible to a small number" of people on the research team (Kashner et al., 2007, p. 394).

Type of Data and Measures

Within the DMP, details of the types of data and the measurement instruments or assessment tools used to capture the data should be well described. This data could be in the form of psychological tests such as the Hamilton Depression Scale (Burnett & Kaplan, 1998), biomarkers such as blood pressure and heart rate, behavioural markers such as movement or vocal patterns, and brain scan data such as fMRI, EEG, and fNRS. More

---

[1] In some trials, it may be important to ensure that the order of multiple questionnaires is standardised or that some items in standardised questionnaires are completed before others. When data is collected and directly entered into the EDCs in real time, EDCs can prevent the assessor from answering questions on the next screen until items on the current screen have been completed.

recently, and as is being used in our MATCH study (Music Attuned Technology Care via eHealth, www.musicattunedcare.com), novel data sources are being used including mobile devices, wearables, in-home sensors, and social media sources (Steinhubl et al., 2015). Other data might relate to feasibility data such as recruitment rates, study completion rates, acceptability of the assessment tools, and acceptability of the intervention; all of these being able to be transformed into numerical data for analysis. For the creative arts therapies, we are unique in including artistic outputs as a type of data that may be considered an "outcome" measure of therapy success. Such data might include a participant composed song (Viega & Baker, 2016) or a piece of art (Berberian et al., 2019), a drama performance (Cook, 2020), and dance/movement (Punkanen et al., 2017).

Data that the research team may also want to collect and analyse may relate directly to the intervention. For example, in some trials, the research team may want to video-record the creative arts therapist's approach and intervention delivery style. This data may be important when the trial is analysing the change process, mechanisms of change, or the impact of the subcomponents of an intervention (De Witte et al., 2021). As such, the video recording *is* the raw data, whereby an analysis of either the therapist, the participant, the creative arts engagement, or all three are analysed using a pre-defined approach to identify the change processes.

Aside from videos being collected *as* data, from time to time video recordings of sessions may be needed so that the researchers can assess treatment adherence and fidelity of the intervention implementation (Baker, Tamplin, Clark, et al., 2019). In this case, video recordings are analysed focusing on what the therapists are doing/not doing, identifying proscribed and prescribed components, and assessing the overall extent to which they are abiding to the study protocol. Both fidelity and adherence to the intervention protocol should be reported in clinical trial publications as part of the trustworthiness and generalisability of the data (see Chapter 8).

Data Collection Methods

As outcomes are regarded as trustworthy when they are based on the collection of consistently high-quality, accurate, complete data, it is imperative that a carefully planned data collection process be developed and described in the DMP. Unreliable or missing data or data collected outside of the pre-defined protocol timepoints is especially problematic when it relates to the primary outcome measure.

The accuracy of data is influenced by several factors that can be partially addressed using an EDC system. Accuracy may be controlled through careful calibration and testing of instruments. Some instruments such as standardised health and wellbeing questionnaires, have already been tested for reliability and validity—but the research team needs to be confident that they are administering the measures as stipulated by the developers of the measures. Further, every participant must be exposed to the same testing conditions and instructions to minimise between participant variability in scores caused by differences in administration. Case Report Forms (electronic or in paper form) can assist in enhancing uniformity of testing conditions (see later this chapter).

Some clinical trials may involve the use of technology that will collect data. The DMP should describe in sufficient detail how to set up, calibrate, and test the data collection tools. In my doctoral studies (Baker, 2007; Baker et al., 2005), I focused on improving the vocal prosody of people with acquired brain injury. To achieve this, I analysed the vocal fundamental frequency and fundamental frequency variability of a set of pre- and post-speaking and singing audio excerpts. These were analysed using KayPENTAX's Multi-Speech™ model 3700 with Real Time Pitch 5121 module. To capture an audio recording that was clean, consistent, and reliable, I recorded participants' voices using a unidirectional microphone headset. This was preferable to a free-standing microphone because people with acquired brain injury may be impulsive and move their heads, thereby increasing the risk of a poor audio quality. To ensure members of the research team were correctly positioning the headset, I provided a detailed set of instructions including pictures.

Technological advances have aided data collection making it more cost-effective and feasible. In the creative arts therapies, Experience Sampling Methods (sometimes referred to as Ecological Momentary Assessment) enable data collection of participants thoughts, feelings, behaviours, or contexts at any time (for example Holt, 2020). Data can be collected at the same time of day or at a random time of day, dependent upon the study aims and outcomes of interest. It has been suggested that such approaches minimise bias stemming from psychological assessment measures (Larson & Csikszentmihalyi, 2014) and can enable continuous monitoring of wellbeing. There are several ways of setting up Experience

Sampling Methods. Participants can be sent an automated phone text message asking them to respond to key questions, or a mobile application downloaded onto their phone can initiate notifications directing them to respond to questions. Links to online surveys can also be sent either by text message or email. Importantly, like all design features of the study, these should be piloted before final decisions made.

All staff collecting data for a trial (whether its members of the research team or members of an organisation's healthcare team) should be well trained in collecting and recording data. Importantly, there should be a clear audit trail—who collected the data, date, time, all ID numbers of participants, etc. If recordings were changed, the person who made the change needs to document reasons why and this should be verified by another member of the team. This will help prevent opportunities for falsifying data. All these processes and procedures should be included in the DMP.

Data Entry

Data entry is the process whereby data collected is inputted into a database. When paper forms are used, traditionally the data is manually entered into a database so that it is converted into an electronic form. While still commonly used, single manual data entry, where data is only entered once, has been shown to be inferior to double manual data entry. EDC systems (see later in this chapter) can assist in minimising invalid responses, but in the case of double-data entry, EDC systems can automate comparisons so that the any conflicts in data that has been doubly entered is flagged. Two-person data entry is now considered the gold standard but is onerous and resource-heavy (Ohmann et al., 2011). While advisable, double-data entry many not always be feasible, especially when budgets are constrained. Whatever method is chosen, the data always needs to be entered in a way that is identifiable, retrievable, and available when needed.

A challenge for many researchers is what and how to collect personal patient health information in a form that is acceptable (Bowman & Maxwell, 2018). As a rule of thumb, it is important to only collect data that is necessary to meet the study objectives. As an example, capturing date of birth is now regarded as an identifiable set of data that should only be used when necessary. In a study with premature babies, an exact birthdate (and in some cases, time of day) may be needed when the creative arts intervention is tracking changes during a period of fast developmental change. Conversely, in my studies of older people living with dementia (Baker, Bloska, et al., 2019), it is only necessary to capture age in years, not actual date year of birth. Other common identifiers are names, addresses, phone numbers, email addresses, social security (or equivalent) numbers, medical record numbers, drivers' licences, and photographs (Bowman & Maxwell, 2018). If these are needed, such data should be kept separate to the database containing health data as there could be a strong risk of identification.

Data Security

In the DMP, procedures for maintaining the security of the data are important not just for the protection of participants' need for privacy, but to protect the integrity of the data. The data must be secure and compliant with any local and international legal obligations. Processes to monitor adherence and data security policies for accessing, reviewing, modifying, or deleting data need to be described in detail in the DMP. All members of the research team need to be familiar with the policy and abide by it. It is usual that the principal investigator is ultimately responsible for the data security.

When undertaking a collaborative research project involving two or more organisations, usually one organisation will "own" the database and is therefore responsible for storing and managing research data. This is normally stipulated in a contractual agreement with all organisations. Several strategies can be adopted to secure data such as password protected databases or filing systems. Most universities have secure cloud options for storing data and have their own individual policies and procedures for storage and access. Becoming familiar with those policies and procedures early on in the project planning phase will enable the research team to set up the data security processes from the outset.

Working internationally can present some challenges when it comes to data storage and security. The General Data Protection Regulation (GDPR, 2016), published by the European Parliament and Council of the European Union and made mandatory across Europe from May 2018, outlines the regulations and practices around data protection. Regardless of the location of the administering organisation,[2] any study involving a European country will need to ensure it abides by GDPR regulations. Outside the European Union, many other countries such as Turkey, Mauritius, Chile, Japan, Brazil, South Korea, Argentina, and Kenya have adopted GDPR regulations. The GDPR was established to enhance an individuals' control and rights over their personal data, including their right to what can be collected and privacy.

Data Cleaning and Quality Control

All research projects should have data cleaning processes in place to improve the quality of the data set. Data cleaning refers to detecting and modifying, replacing, or deleting incomplete, incorrect, improperly formatted, duplicated, or irrelevant records, otherwise referred to as dirty data, within a database (Allen, 2017; Love et al., 2021). Undertaking data cleaning will result in a trustworthy final data set for statistical or qualitative analysis.

There are a few basic steps that are helpful to consider when cleaning your data (Van den Broeck et al., 2005). Step 1 involves removing duplicate data. When importing data from multiple places, there is a likelihood that the same data may be inputted more than once into the database, especially if some of the data is automated. The second step involves fixing structural errors such as editing incorrect naming conventions. For example when reviewing the database, it may be observed that art therapy, "AThep" and AT (art therapy)(which indicate the same thing, or "NA", "N/A", and "not applicable" appear. When cleaning the database, items should be labelled in the same way. Once these have been fixed, there is an important step in filtering out unwanted outliers. Outliers can be the result of an error in data entry. Step 4 concerns the handling of missing data (see Chapter 9). The final step involves validating the data. Here the data is reviewed to assess whether the data is plausible and follows the rules for each field.

---

[2] Where several local, national, or international institutions are part of a large trial, the administering organisation is the university, hospital, or research institute that leads the study; the organisation who ultimately takes responsibility for the project.

The data manager (see Chapter 4) is a specialist who will check the data at regular timepoints whose priority is to ensure that the data entered in the database falls within an expected range. As alluded to earlier, if there are any outliers, this could signal that there is an input error that should be checked and if necessary, corrected. There are some examples however, where outliers are correct values. For example, if the age of a person is entered into the database as 118, this would be considered well above the usual age of human and should be questioned. The entry may be correct—there are plenty of centenarians these days—but the unusual entry might trigger the data manager to double check the accuracy.

EDC systems can be structured to reduce the workload associated with data cleaning. For example, rather than typing in a response into a free field, the EDC system can be formatted to include dropdown menus or radio buttons with a given set of options. Similarly, items can be set up to prevent entries of numbers outside the valid range of scores. In our HOMESIDE study, radio buttons were used to record the relationship of the caregiver to the person with dementia they were caring for—partner/spouse, son, daughter, sibling, and friend. Similarly, the calculation of the total scores on some measures were automated, again reducing the risk of human error. Such formats are become increasingly important for outcome measures where some items have reverse scoring. The system can be set to automatically reverse those specific items, thereby eliminating errors made in calculating scores by a data-entry person.

Case Study. Cleaning of Audio Data for Speech Analysis. Sometimes electronically captured data needs to be cleaned so it can be accurately analysed. In studies I have been involved in which have used recorded audio data to analyse changes in vocal abilities of people with acquired brain injury and people with Parkinson's disease (Baker et al., 2005; Elefant et al., 2012; Tamplin et al., 2019, 2020), we have utilised various software to measure the characteristics of the audio recordings. One such software mentioned earlier was KayPENTAX's Multi-Speech™ model 3700 with Real Time Pitch 5121 module. It analyses volume (decibels), average pitch of speaking voice (fundamental frequency), and prosody (variability in the frequency), as well as glottal event markers, formant history, spectrogram, and energy. While this process is automated, the accuracy of the analysis can easily be affected by audio contamination. When audio data is captured in a clinical setting as opposed to a soundproofed studio, it is likely that extraneous sounds such as a door squeak, a bird chirping outside, or the sound of wind gusts can be heard within the audio sample and are thus at risk of inappropriately becoming a part of the audio analysis. It is possible to calibrate the software to minimise the impact of such contamination. In my doctoral studies, my trial demanded considerable calibration of the software. Let us take the sample I recorded below of a male who spoke a simple sentence into a microphone—Fig. 7.1. The figure clearly shows how the frequencies highlighted by the circles, were extraneous sounds in the sample that did not reflect the frequency of the participant's voice. Figure 7.2 highlights the results of the data analysis processed by the software for this sample.

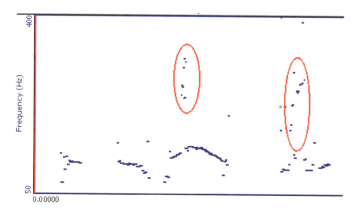

Fig. 7.1 Sample of contour prior to adjustment to frequency levels

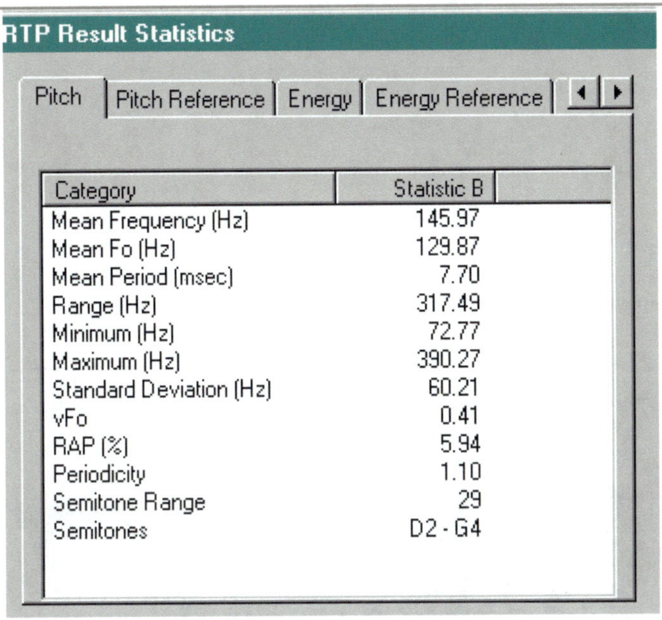

RTP Result Statistics	
Pitch	Pitch Reference	Energy	Energy Reference		

Category	Statistic B
Mean Frequency (Hz)	145.97
Mean Fo (Hz)	129.87
Mean Period (msec)	7.70
Range (Hz)	317.49
Minimum (Hz)	72.77
Maximum (Hz)	390.27
Standard Deviation (Hz)	60.21
vFo	0.41
RAP (%)	5.94
Periodicity	1.10
Semitone Range	29
Semitones	D2 - G4

Fig. 7.2 Results of contour analysis pre-frequency adjustment

Using the cleaning functions within MultiSpeech, I was able to "clean" the data by applying a series of instructions to limit the range of frequencies that were able to be analysed, a so called "smoothing of the data". The resultant effect is that of a clean audio signal free from the outliers seen in Fig. 7.1. Figure 7.3 illustrates the frequencies to be analysed in the same audio sample following the smoothing of the data. This resultant outcome is that I feel more confident that I am actually analysing the true effects of the music intervention—this calibration improved research integrity. When comparing the analysis of data automated by the software in Figs. 7.2 with 7.4, the mean fundamental frequency decreased from 129.87 Hz to119.40 Hz, highlighting how a cleaner signal can change the output.

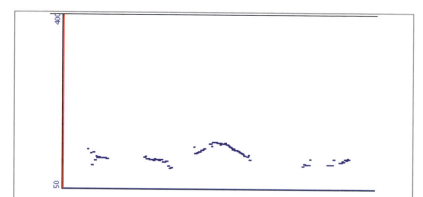

Fig. 7.3 Sample of contour post adjustment to frequency levels

RTP Result Statistics — Pitch	
Category	Statistic B
Mean Frequency (Hz)	121.05
Mean Fo (Hz)	119.40
Mean Period (msec)	8.38
Range (Hz)	51.75
Minimum (Hz)	92.84
Maximum (Hz)	144.59
Standard Deviation (Hz)	14.35
vFo	0.12
RAP (%)	1.30
Periodicity	1.11
Semitone Range	8
Semitones	F#2 - D3

Fig. 7.4 Results of contour analysis post-frequency adjustment

Case Report Forms

Case report forms (CRFs) are documents that are either in electronic or in paper form that are used to record all protocol-required information (Fleischmann et al., 2017). CRFs are very helpful documents for keeping track of what data needs to be collected, the order, and how they should be administered. CRFs are developed for every component of the trial from expressions of interest, screening phone calls, plain language statements and consent forms, baseline and follow-up data, fidelity checklists for assessors, and those delivering the interventions. These forms often contain "scripts" which enable the person designated to collect that data, to implement it consistent manner. This minimises the impact of potential variations (and therefore another factor impacting the findings) in administration of assessments and implementation of creative arts therapies programs. CRFs, whether electronic or in paper form, should be checked, verified, and dated by one member of the research team to avoid members tampering with the data and falsifying information later.

Data Access: Roles and Responsibilities

Who, when, and what data is accessed by members of the team needs to be carefully considered, well described in the DMP, and systems set up so that accidental access to data does not occur. Inappropriate access can threaten data security. Additionally, accidental access by the wrong members of the team may compromise the integrity of the project. For example, researchers involved in collecting data related to outcome measures should not have access to data where randomisation or intervention allocation data is detailed. This will reduce the likelihood of allocation unmasking. This is especially important in a cluster randomised controlled trial whereby if one participant's allocation is unmasked, it means the data for the whole cluster is unmasked.

When leading international trials, separating data access between countries may also be necessary, especially if data sharing is violating international data security standards. This means that each country should not have access to each other's data until it can be presented in a de-identifiable format.

Utilising the functions within EDC systems can assist in controlling data access. Data-access groups are commonly used to help multiple groups of researchers access only the parts of the database that are relevant to their role. To illustrate, our HOMESIDE project had several data-access groups. There were data-access groups for the principal investigator and data manager who had access to almost the entire data set (Table 7.2). The statistician and health economist had access to certain data that was relevant to them, and then we had data-access groups for each country (Germany, Poland, the United Kingdom, Norway, and Australian teams only had access to data for participants in their respective countries). However, within each country, there were further data-access restrictions dependent upon each individual team member's role. Country leaders (the chief investigator for each country) were able to export data and create reports pertaining to data from their own country, verify and lock database entries made by their respective research teams, and enter data into the database as needed. Each country had an assessor team—researchers who collected the outcome measures data and who were masked to participant allocation. They were given access to view and edit entries in the database only for the REDCap modules related to assessment. Similarly, the interventionists within each country had view and edit entries related to modules which related to the intervention data. Examples will be described later in this chapter.

Data Storage

The DMP needs to detail how the data will be stored during the trial and for archiving post-trial. Several cloud-based data storage software packages are now available which can accommodate large amounts of clinical trial data. Many university and healthcare organisations make use of Microsoft Office 365 cloud-based approaches including the use of OneDrive and Sharepoint. EDC systems such as REDCap and Open Clinica are also increasingly used and stored in highly secure systems managed by the Information Technology teams at each institution. Other systems such as Mediaflux can manage both structured and unstructured data. For example, in a project collecting large amounts of video material of participants participating in a creative arts therapy session/s, Mediaflux can be a highly secure means to store very large media files.

Table 7.2 HOMESIDE REDCap Roles

	Principal investigator/data manager	Country leader	Statistician/health economist	Assessor	Interventionist
Data Export—Full data set	X	X			
Add/Edit Reports	X	X			
Statistics and Charts	X	X			
Logging	X	X	X		
File Repository	X	X	X		
Randomisation—Dashboard	X	X	X		
Randomisation—Randomise		X			
Data Quality—Create and edit rules	X	X	X		
Data Quality—Execute Rules	X	X			
REDCap Mobile App allows use to—To collect data offline	X	X		X	X
Create Records	X	X		X	
Rename Records	X	X			
Record Locking Customisation	X	X			
Locking/Unlocking Records	X	X			
Data-Entry Rights					
Expressions of Interest/Screening (all modules)	$X^{\#}$	$X^{\#}$		$X^{\#}$	
Assessment (all modules)	$X^{\#}$	$X^{\#}$	X^{*}	$X^{\#}$	
Randomisation	$X^{\#}$	$X^{\#}$	X^{*}		
Intervention (all modules) and Diary	$X^{\#}$	$X^{\#}$	X^{*}		$X^{\#}$
Fidelity Checklist (Assessment's modules)	$X^{\#}$	$X^{\#}$	X^{*}	$X^{\#}$	
Fidelity Checklist (Intervention's modules)	$X^{\#}$	$X^{\#}$	X^{*}		$X^{\#}$

X = full access, X^{*} = read only access, $X^{\#}$ = view and edit access

Study Participant Monitoring

A reliable and systematic system of tracking participant flow throughout the study period is one the most important tasks of data monitoring. The data monitoring system should enable the research team to track a participant's progress from the initial expression of interest to participate, through to final follow-up assessment, and this process should be consistent with the Consolidated Standards for Reporting Trials (CONSORT, 2010). The CONSORT is a set of recommendations for reporting of randomised controlled trials including its design, methods, results, and conclusions. The CONSORT group created a 25-item checklist and flow diagram which provides guidance for the reporting of study enrolment, retention, monitoring, and the derivation of analytic data sets. The participant data collected and monitored through the study should enable this diagram to be simply and accurately completed.

To derive the participant data set, the EDC system is designed so that the following can be captured in the final data set:

- *Screening/Recruitment*: the number of potential participants screened for inclusion/exclusion criteria and reasons for exclusion. Data captured will clearly signal that only eligible participants are enrolled.
- *Discontinuation of Intervention*: At times, participants may discontinue the intervention but choose to remain in the study. The system should capture when, if, and why the intervention was discontinued. For example, change in family circumstances, dislike of the intervention (but not an adverse event), etc. Participants may remain in the study and included in the intention-to-treat sample, or even the per-protocol sample if they had completed the minimum intervention adherence.
- *Withdrawals*: The system should capture when, if, and why the participant withdrew from the project. This could be due to an adverse event related to participant in the intervention or the assessment of outcome measures, or for other reasons. In such circumstances, no further data will be collected from the participants but, dependent upon the trial protocol, their data to that withdrawal point may be included in the intention-to-treat analysis or per-protocol analysis.

- *Adverse Events*: Every DMP should contain a protocol for the reporting and documentation of any adverse event, serious adverse event, and deaths.

DATA SHARING AND LONG-TERM PRESERVATION

Each DMP must contain a policy and procedure for data sharing and long-term preservation of data. The description should include how and when data will be shared and whether there are any restrictions to data sharing or embargo. The plan should also include how data will be selected for preservation and where the data will be preserved long term, for example in a data repository[3] or archive. The plan should also include the methods or software tools that will be needed to access the data.

In addition to the long-term preservation of the data set, the DMP needs to include descriptions of who will have access to unprocessed (raw) data. It is important to determine this not just from a privacy aspect, but also from the perspective intellectual property, especially if the research involves commercialisation potential.[4]

> *Case Study. MATCH, Intellectual Property, and Commercialisation.* Our MATCH project is developing, testing, and refining a music technology that aimed to regulate the behavioural and psychological symptoms of dementia as well as embedding within it, a robust family and professional career training program. As with all publicly funded research projects in Australia (and in many places around the globe), it is a requirement to make data available for reuse when appropriate. As we were intending to commercialise the MATCH eHealth solution either for profit or as a social enterprise, we needed to discern which data was commercially sensitive and should not be placed in the public domain. This included a careful assessment of what data could be potentially used by any competitors to "get into the market" faster than our team. After a thorough assessment, we identified three levels of data access:

---

[3] A data repository refers to a data storage entity where data is stored for analytical or reporting purposes. The purpose of keeping a repository is so that certain data for a population can be mined for greater insight or for specific reporting.

[4] Intellectual property and commercialisation are explored in more detail in Chapter 11.

1. Open access data refers to the data that is permissible to be accessed in a de-identified format. Here, this data did not relate to commercial project outcomes or impact benefit or competitiveness of the research outputs, including specific structure and mechanisms of the eHealth intervention that may benefit the public. This may include data relating to participants with dementias' responses to different types of music or to their use of technology.
2. Restricted access data refers to data that will be restricted for a fixed period. In our study, data that may be confidential and impact our market competitiveness will not be shared prior to the public launch of our eHealth solution. The choice of data in this category was discussed by senior members of the team all the way through the trial and determined by the principal investigator with input from the relevant chief investigators, as well as informed by the university's knowledge and technology transfer experts.
3. Confidential data refers to data that will never be shared due to the risk of competitors using the data to advance the development of their own commercial product. In our study, this data was specific to the eHealth solution including the source code, novel interactions between software and hardware, and user responses to specific aspects of the project. This data was to be kept confidential and appropriately stored.

Monitoring and Reporting

Within the DMP, there may be a section that details the frequency and types of reporting that will be conducted throughout the trial. The frequency of monitoring reports will depend on the scope of the trial, its complexity, and timeline. For example, in a 12-month art therapy trial, measuring the impact of a brief art therapy program on child pre-operative anxiety and pain, frequent monitoring of adverse events may be needed (possibly a review every month). Conversely, a three-year dance/movement therapy project which is evaluating the long-term impact of a program on grief and trauma with people who have successfully recovered from breast cancer treatment, monitoring may be needed less frequently. Reports generated can provide the team with quick and clear snapshots of how the project is tracking according to its timelines and deliverables.

Developing an Electronic Data Capture System for Your Trial

As mentioned earlier, EDC systems are a useful way to manage large sets of complex data and enabling the research team to track participants through the study period. Importantly, every trial should have a purposefully designed database to meet that project's specific data collection, monitoring, and analytic needs. This next section of the chapter outlines the process of developing an EDC system and illustrates these with some screenshots of the user interface.

Overview of the EDC System Development Process

There are four stages to the development of an EDC system. The first is to establish the database requirements. During this phase, the research teams begin by meeting with the information scientist(s) and those developing the database, to determine the requirements specific to that project. In addition to mapping out the design and what data needs to be collected, the team should discuss who will need to access/edit the data, how data will be secured, and the processes needed to validate/lock data (Harris et al., 2009). The research team will be asked to complete an excel spreadsheet where metadata information needs to be added. Metadata will include information such as a field name, end-user label, data type, and data range for each measurement included in each case report form.

In the second development phase, the database team converts the metadata into a set of database tables. Once the research team are satisfied that they have the data requirements needed, the database development moves to a "release and test" phase where the research team can test the prototype of the database. During this phase, the research team are given instructions to test the database, recommending revisions as needed. If some of the modules within the database are going to be forwarded to participants for remote completion such as an online survey or questionnaire (as was the case when we implemented our MATCH "face and content validity" study), then part of the testing will include exploring and piloting layout options. Modifications can be made as necessary. Once the prototype has been thoroughly tested, and the research team has signed off that it is ready for implementation within the study, the project database is deployed for use.

Database User Interface

The database user interface can be somewhat daunting when first logging in an viewing it. However, if researchers take time to explore its functionality, they will soon become comfortable using it, and will recognise how much faster and easier it is to access data, identify missing data, and view patterns when compared with clunky excel spreadsheets. For example, every month the five HOMESIDE country team leaders and myself met to discuss details the progress of the trial. Until recruitment ended in June 2022, each monthly meeting had one part of it devoted to discussing recruitment numbers and strategies to boost recruitment. The database enabled the data manager to quickly generate reports that detailed enrolments right up to the day of the meeting. This provided a current and accurate picture of recruitment since the previous meeting so that the success of implemented strategies could be reviewed and discussed.

When first logging on to a database in REDCap, the left-hand menu lists several options and functions of the database (Fig. 7.5).[5] There are four main sections in the database. First, there is the Project Home and Design section which provides information on the structure of the database, the codebook and dictionary. This section is what the database manager uses to create and manage the project database. The second section of the database comprises the data collection tools. Here, every CRF that the research team developed has been converted into an electronic module so that the relevant member of the team can enter the data into the system. In Fig. 7.5, data collection modules available include expressions of interest, COVID-19 screening questions, consent forms, baseline assessments, etc.

Figure 7.6 illustrates what one of these modules might look like to a participant who receives a link to complete a questionnaire. This module includes a series of Likert scale statements using radio buttons rather than free-text responses. Once completed by participants, their responses are directly deposited into the database alongside all the other data collected about participants with this same identification number.

Under the Project Applications tab, are a collection of tools that enable the research team to explore the database. Perhaps the most important

---

[5] What database users will see will be dependent upon their data-access rights (for example as displayed in Table 7.2).

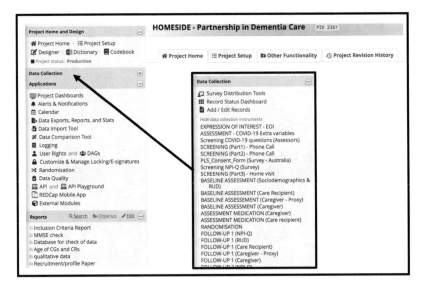

Fig. 7.5 HOMESIDE REDCap database home page

function the principal investigator will utilise during the trial is the dashboard. The dashboard enables the principal researcher to view which of the data collection modules have been completed for each participant. The dashboards' default position is to display the completion of all modules; however, it is possible to filter the database so that only certain modules are explored. Our HOMESIDE dashboard has been set up so that the principal investigator can view all data via the default dashboard, or (1) just all the expressions of interest, (2) all baseline/follow-up modules for the main outcome measures, (3) all fidelity checks of intervention videos, (4) all assessment data, (5) all intervention data, (6) all qualitative data, and the (7) randomisation data as illustrated in the dropdown menu in Fig. 7.7. It is also possible to filter by data-access group. In Fig. 7.7, the baseline/follow-up dashboard has been loaded just for the data collected from the Polish research team. Each dyad (person living with dementia and their family carer) has an identification number as listed in the very left column. Then, each of the data collection modules that are displayed in this dashboard are listed across the top. The green radio buttons indicate the modules that have been completed for each dyad. Here, dyad PL001 has completed the baseline

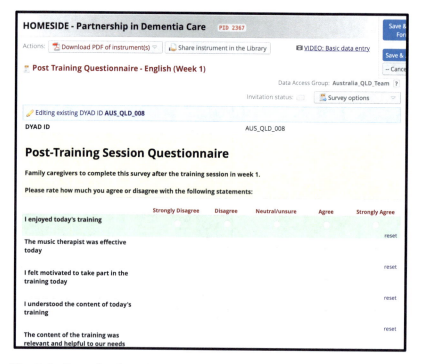

Fig. 7.6 Example of a HOMESIDE data collection module

data (including the main outcome measure NPI-Q) and the two follow-up measures. Notably, there were no adverse events reported by assessors or those interventionists providing the interventions.

Finally, the last section of the database enables the research team to create reports for exporting. This data may be needed by the trial steering committee or data safety monitoring board (see Chapter 3), or just by the trial management group who will periodically want to review the data set.

Conclusion

Developing a good database and having well-defined policies and processes in place to collect, store, manage, and monitor data places the research team in the best position to arrive with a reliable data set at the end of data collection. The larger and the more complex the trial

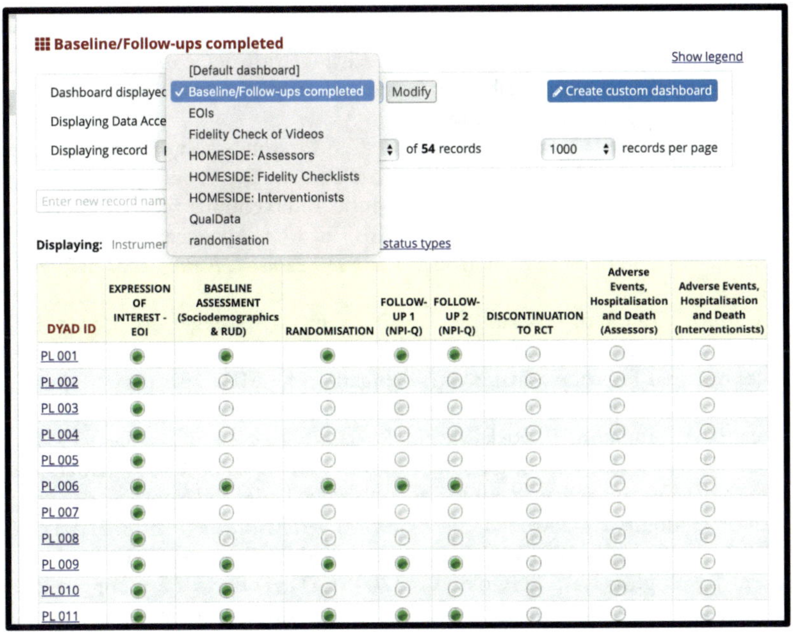

Fig. 7.7 HOMESIDE Baseline/Follow-ups REDCap Dashboard

becomes, the more important it is to have a system which keeps the data organised and easily accessible. It is imperative that the team takes the time to develop, test, and review the database before moving it from the development to production phase.

References

Allen, M. (2017). Data cleaning. In M. Allen (Ed.), *The Sage encyclopaedia of communication research methods* (pp. 338–339). https://doi.org/10.4135/9781483381411.n126

Baker, F. (2007). Using voice analysis software to analyse the sung and spoken voice. In T. Wosch & T. Wigram (Eds.), *Microanalysis: Methods, techniques and applications in music therapy for clinicians, researchers, educators and students* (pp. 101–113). Jessica Kingsley Publishers.

Baker, F. A., Bloska, J., Stensæth, K., Wosch, T., Bukowska, A., Braat, S., Sousa, T., Tamplin, J., Clark, I. N., Lee, Y.-E. C., Clarke, P., Lautenschlager,

N., & Odell-Miller, H. (2019). HOMESIDE: A home-based family caregiver-delivered music intervention for people living with dementia: Protocol of a randomised controlled trial. *British Medical Journal Open.* https://doi.org/10.1136/bmjopen-2019-031332

Baker, F. A., Lee, Y.-E. C., Sousa, T. V., Stretton-Smith, P. A., Tamplin, J., Sveinsdottir, V., Geretsegger, M., Wake, J. D., Assmus, J., & Gold, C. (2022). Clinical effectiveness of Music Interventions for Dementia and Depression in Elderly care (MIDDEL) in the Australian cohort: pragmatic cluster-randomised controlled trial. *The Lancet Healthy Longevity, 3*(3), e153–e165.

Baker, F. A., Tamplin, J., Clark, I., Lee, Y.-E. C., Geretsegger, M., & Gold, C. (2019). Treatment fidelity in a music therapy multi-site cluster randomized control trial for people living with dementia: The MIDDEL project. *Journal of Music Therapy.* https://doi.org/10.1093/jmt/thy023

Baker, F. A., Tamplin, J., Rickard, N., Ponsford, J., New, P., & Lee, Y.-E. C. (2019). A therapeutic songwriting intervention to promote reconstruction of self-concept and enhance wellbeing following brain and spinal cord injury: Pilot randomised controlled trial. *Clinical Rehabilitation.* https://doi.org/10.1177/0123456789123456. First Published 22 February 2019.

Baker, F., Wigram, T., & Gold, C. (2005). The effects of a song-singing programme on the affective speaking intonation of people with traumatic brain injury. *Brain Injury, 19*(7), 519–528.

Berberian, M., Walker, M. S., & Kaimal, G. (2019). "Master My Demons": Art therapy montage paintings by active-duty military service members with traumatic brain injury and post-traumatic stress. *Medical Humanities, 45*(4), 353–360. https://doi.org/10.1136/medhum-2018-011493

Bowman, M. A., & Maxwell, R. A. (2018). A beginner's guide to avoiding Protected Health Information (PHI) issues in clinical research—With how-to's in REDCap data management software. *Journal of Biomedical Informatics, 85*, 49. https://doi.org/10.1016/j.jbi.2018.07.008

Burnett, P. C., & Kaplan, B. J. (1998). *Revised Hamilton rating scale for depression.* American Psychological Association.

CONSORT. (2010). *Consolidated Standards for Reporting Trials.* CONSORT Group. http://www.consort-statement.org. Accessed 25 October 2021.

Cook, A. (2020). Using an inclusive therapeutic theatre production to teach self-advocacy skills in young people with disabilities. *The Arts in Psychotherapy, 71*, 101715. https://doi.org/10.1016/j.aip.2020.101715

De Witte, M., Orkibi, H., Zarate, R., Karkou, V., Sanjani, N., Malhotra, B., Ho, R. T. H., Kaimal, G., Baker, F. A., & Koch, S. C. (2021). Identifying mechanisms of change for psychological health outcomes in the creative arts therapies. A scoping review. *Frontiers in Psychology, 12*, 678397. https://doi.org/10.3389/fpsyg.2021.678397. Published online 15 July 2021.

Elefant, C., Baker, F., Lotan, M., Lagersen, S., & Skeie, G. O. (2012). Effect of group music therapy on vocal ability and singing in individuals with Parkinson's disease—A feasibility research. *Journal of Music Therapy, 49*(3), 278–302.

European Parliament and Council of the European Union. (2016). *General Data Protection Regulation,* L119, COM/2012/010 final—2012/0010 (COD). https://gdpr-info.eu. Accessed 22 October 20221.

Fleischmann, R., Decker, A.-M., Kraft, A., Mai, K., & Schmidt, S. (2017). Mobile electronic versus paper case report forms in clinical trials: A randomized controlled trial. *BMC Medical Research Methodology, 17*(1), 1–10. https://doi.org/10.1186/s12874-017-0429-y

Harris, P. A., Taylor, R., Thielke, R., Payne, J., Gonzalez, N., & Conde, J. G. (2009). Research electronic data capture (REDCap)—A metadata-driven methodology and workflow process for providing translational research informatics support. *Journal of Biomedical Informatics, 42*(2), 377–381. https://doi.org/10.1016/j.jbi.2008.08.010

Holt, N. J. (2020). Tracking momentary experience in the evaluation of arts-on-prescription services: Using mood changes during art workshops to predict global wellbeing change. *Perspectives in Public Health, 140*(5), 270–276.

ICH. (2021). *Guideline for good clinical practice.* International Council for Harmonisation of Technical Requirements for Pharmaceuticals for Human Use. https://database.ich.org/sites/default/files/ICH_E6-R3_GCP-Principles_Draft_2021_0419.pdf. Accessed 25 October 2021.

Kashner, T. M., Hinson, R., Holland, G. J., Mickey, D. D., Hoffman, K., Lind, L., Johnson, L. D., Chang, B. K., Golden, R. M., & Henley, S. S. (2007). A data accounting system for clinical investigators. *Journal of the American Medical Informatics Association, 4*, 394–396.

Larson, R., & Csikszentmihalyi, M. (2014). The experience sampling method. In I. M. Csikszentmihalyi (Ed.), *Flow and the foundations of positive psychology* (pp. 21–34). Springer.

Love, S. B., Yorke-Edwards, V., Diaz-Montana, C., Murray, M. L., Masters, L., Gabriel, M., Joffe, N., & Sydes, M. R. (2021). Making a distinction between data cleaning and central monitoring in clinical trials. *Clinical Trials, 18*(3), 386–388. https://doi.org/10.1177/1740774520976617

Molloy, S. F., & Henley, P. (2016). Monitoring clinical trials: A practical guide. *Tropical Medicine and International Health, 21*(12), 1602. https://doi.org/10.1111/tmi.12781

Ohmann, C., Kuchinke, W., Canham, S., Lauritsen, J., Salas, N., Schade-Brittinger, C., Wittenberg, M., McPherson, G., McCourt, J., Gueyffier, F., Lorimer, A., & Torres, F. (2011). Standard requirements for GCP-compliant data management in multinational clinical trials. *Trials, 12*(1), 85.

Punkanen, M., Saarikallio, S., Leinonen, O., Forsblom, A., Kulju, J., & Luck, G. (2017). Emotions in motion: Depression in dance-movement and dance-movement in treatment of depression. In V. Karkou, S. Oliver, & S. Lycouris (Eds.), *The Oxford handbook of dance and wellbeing*. https://doi.org/10.1093/oxfordhb/9780199949298.013.58

Steinhubl, S. R., Muse, E. D., & Topol, E. J. (2015). The emerging field of mobile health. *Science Translational Medicine, 7*(283), 283rv3.

Tamplin, J., Marigliani, C., Morris, M., Baker, F. A., & Vogel, A. P. (2019). A controlled trial of therapeutic group singing to improve speech and voice in Parkinson's disease. *Neurorehabilitation and Neural Repair, 33*(6), 453–463.

Tamplin, J., Morris, M., Marigliani, C., Baker, F. A., Noff, G., & Vogel, A. P. (2020). ParkinSong: Outcomes of a 12-month controlled trial of therapeutic singing groups in Parkinson's disease. *Journal of Parkinson's Disease*. https://doi.org/10.3233/JPD-191838

United States Department of Health and Human Services (HHS). (2018, March). *Good Clinical Practice: Integrated Addendum to ICH E6(R1)*. Guidance for Industry, OMB Control No. 0910-0843. https://www.fda.gov/downloads/Drugs/Guidances/UCM464506.pdf

Van den Broeck, J., Cunningham, S. A., Eeckels, R., & Herbst, K. (2005). Data cleaning: Detecting, diagnosing, and editing data abnormalities. *PLoS Medicine, 2*(10), e267. https://doi.org/10.1371/journal.pmed.0020267

Viega, M. D., & Baker, F. A. (2016). What's in a song? Combining analytical and arts-based analysis for songs created by songwriters with neurodisabilities. *Nordic Journal of Music Therapy*. https://doi.org/10.1080/08098131.2016.1205651

World Medical Association. (2018). *WMA Declaration of Helsinki*. World Medical Association. https://www.wma.net/policies-post/wma-declaration-of-helsinki-ethical-principles-for-medical-research-involving-human-subjects/. First Accessed 25 October 2021.

Zozus, M. N., Kahn, M. G., & Weiskopf, N. G. (2019). Data quality in clinical research. In R. Richesson & J. Andrews (Eds.), *Clinical research informatics. Health informatics*. Springer. https://doi.org/10.1007/978-3-319-98779-8_11

CHAPTER 8

Development, Measurement, and Validation of Intervention Fidelity

WHAT IS FIDELITY AND WHY IS IT IMPORTANT?

Historically, the word fidelity has been used to describe being "faithful" to a person, cause, or belief, as well as the extent to which an action or item is copied or reproduced. In the context of research, intervention fidelity (sometimes referred to as treatment fidelity, implementation fidelity, research integrity, and adherence to protocol) bridges both these concepts and is defined as the processes used to determine whether an intervention and study implementation more generally is delivered as intended by those who developed it (Dusenbury et al., 2003). Determining and recording the extent of intervention fidelity within a clinical trial captures important information to help the researchers understand why an intervention may or may not have influenced its intended health outcome (Ginsburg et al., 2021) and improves research integrity. In other words, could an effect (or non-effect) be the result of intended or unintended modifications to the intervention protocol.

In drawing indisputable conclusions about the effectiveness of complex interventions (internal validity), and to facilitate research replication and generalisability (external validity), it is important that systems to safeguard and accurately assess fidelity are put in place prior to commencement of a study (Bellg et al., 2004; Borrelli et al., 2005; Walton et al., 2017). When fidelity is not considered in the design, planning, and implementation of a trial, there is a very real risk that outcomes of the trial are caused by factors not related to the planned intervention (Ginsburg et al., 2021). Many research studies within the creative arts therapies test the implementation of highly complex interventions where there are often multiple interacting components. Such complexities present challenges in developing and assessing fidelity processes (Walton et al., 2017); however, it is for these very reasons that fidelity needs to be measured (Carrol et al., 2007).

Fidelity strategies can assist in reducing the possibility of Type I, Type II, and Type III errors. Type I errors (false positive) occur when a trial has results that suggest an intervention is significantly effective when it is not. Type I errors can occur for example, when proscribed elements[1] of the intervention are added or other components are omitted (Borrelli et al., 2005; Ginsburg et al., 2021). Here, monitoring fidelity will help protect the possibility that it was some other factor rather than the intervention itself, that was responsible for the health improvements noted. Type II errors (false negatives) are those errors that occur when the trial failed to detect a significant effect when one exists. Similar to Type I errors, Type II errors can occur from adding or omitting components to the therapy, which subsequently lead to not detecting an intervention effect (Ginsburg et al., 2021; Moncher & Prinz, 1991). Type III errors occur when the researchers get the right answer to the wrong question (Carroll et al., 2007). It is possible that the intervention was not delivered with consistently high quality; therefore, it is possible the intervention is effective but was not delivered to a standard high enough to effect a change (Feely et al., 2018). There are several approaches to safeguarding fidelity that will be discussed later in this chapter.

> *Case Example. Dance/Movement Therapy.* Consider this scenario—a dance/movement therapy trial is examining a manual-based group intervention protocol for culturally sensitive short-term dance/movement therapy, to determine its effect on bodily and psychological perceptions in Ultra- Orthodox Jewish women (Suskin & Al-Yagon, 2020).

---

[1] Proscribed elements of an intervention are those that are prohibited either because they are (a) a feature of the comparative intervention, (b) that they introduce an element of an intervention that may counter the intended effect, or (c) the outcome produced (positive or negative) may be result of the introduction of that element rather than the elements that are prescribed.

> While not a randomised controlled trial with a control or comparative active condition, the pre-post effects were evaluated using standardised psychological measurements. To reach the sample size of 47, the authors implemented three separate groups using a manualised approach. The manualised approach was used to promote fidelity and to ensure that each of three groups received an intervention that was comparable.

> *Case Example. Music Therapy.* In our MIDDEL music intervention study with residential care home residents with dual diagnosis of depression and dementia (MIDDEL, Baker, Tamplin, et al., 2019, Gold et al., 2019, Baker et al., 2022), we tested two different music interventions. Group music therapy (GMT) was delivered in small groups by registered music therapists, and recreational choir singing (RCS) was delivered in larger groups by a community musician. Group music therapy included a more personalised music experiences and the therapist intentionally adopted methods such as singing resident-preferred repertoire, musical attunement and music-stimulated reminiscence with the therapeutic delivery embedding principles of Kitwood's personhood. Conversely, the RCS comprised the singing of familiar songs only. Fidelity measures were put in place to enable that the complexity of each intervention to be captured, documented, and monitored. Additionally, the fidelity measures provided an avenue to ensure that each intervention were sufficiently differentiated as to explain any differences in the outcomes. This will be discussed later in this chapter.

In addition to reducing the risk of Type I, II, and III errors, good fidelity processes can contribute to the strengthening of secondary research—systematic reviews and meta-analyses (Carrol et al., 2007). Here, any missing reporting on fidelity may impact the assessment of heterogeneity between studies. Such a lack of knowledge of heterogeneity may then lead to pooling or aggregating studies inappropriately (Roen et al., 2006). When this occurs, there is the potential to adversely effect the internal validity of the review, and therefore the generalisability and usefulness of the outcomes (Carrol et al., 2007). Poorly monitored fidelity will lessen the credibility and utility of that research.

Reporting of Intervention Fidelity in Creative Arts Therapies Literature

As outlined in the introductory chapter, compared with the entire field of non-pharmacological interventions more broadly, very few creative arts therapy researchers have had the opportunity to implement large-scale clinical trials, supported by adequate funding and infrastructure. Further, unless the novice creative arts therapy researcher has had access to good mentoring, research training, and has been engaged in interdisciplinary collaborative research, very few would have the deep understanding and knowledge about the importance of, and processes needed to establish intervention fidelity in clinical trials. For the first decade of my research career, I certainly fell into this category.

Treatment fidelity is certainly a concept that is beginning to be referenced in creative arts therapies research. Specific creative arts therapy publications that reference the reporting, the importance of, and/or how to implement fidelity strategies is an exception rather than the rule. Robb et al. (2011), Baker, Tamplin, et al. (2019), and Honig and McKinney (2021) all highlight the need for music therapy/music intervention studies to develop and report on intervention fidelity. Robb et al. (2018) found that in the 187 included music intervention clinical trials studies published between 2010–2015, only 20% of studies reported treatment fidelity. Feniger-Schaal and Orkibi (2020), undertook a systematic review of drama therapy research and found that only 10 of the 24 (42%) included studies, reported the degree to which interventions were delivered as per the protocol.

Systematic review of arts-based interventions targeting improved cognition in older adults with mild cognitive impairment (Fong et al., 2021) found that of the 11 RCTs included in the review, 3 were at high risk of insufficient intervention reporting, and a further 8 of some concern. While there was no specific reference to adherence or fidelity as such, one can imply that it was assessed through the study quality appraisal process. Of the five quality appraisal categories, the category of reporting of deviations from intended interventions was the only category where there was some risk or high risk of bias. A full systematic review of the quality of intervention studies across art therapy and dance movement therapy which would highlight the trends in reporting fidelity, have yet to be undertaken, but it is likely that with the emergence of more and more clinical trials protocols published in journals and in clinical trials registry (for example Chan et al., 2021), the increasing level of awareness of the importance of intervention fidelity, and increasing numbers of more highly funded trials (which is needed to sufficiently resource fidelity), that reporting of fidelity will increase.

Conceptual Frameworks of Fidelity

Fidelity conceptual frameworks fall into two broad approaches. The first concerns the engagement between the study participant and the interventionist who is providing the manualised intervention, and the second offers a "broader view, and incorporates organisational variables" (Feely et al., 2018). I am not going to discuss the latter. At the participant-therapist level, there are four main dimensions of fidelity—adherence and exposure (dose) to the intervention, quality of the intervention delivery, component differentiation, and participant responsiveness (Carrol et al., 2007; Proctor et al., 2011). Let's examine each in turn.

Intervention Adherence

Adherence is defined as the extent to which the interventions were delivered as intended (Mihalic, 2004) and has been considered the essential "bottom-line measurement" of implementation fidelity (Carrol et al., 2007). Adherence has a content-related component and an exposure component. The content fidelity relates to the extent to which the content of the intervention is present in the therapy. Within the creative arts therapies, this could be content within a single session, or over the whole program. The exposure component refers to the extent to which the participant was "exposed" to the intervention, or what is sometimes referred to as "dose". It measures how much of the intervention was delivered. For example, how many sessions of therapy were implemented, attended, how frequently, and the duration of the sessions. Therefore, adherence by exposure is the extent to which a participants' participation maps against what was proposed in the protocol. When the intervention is assessed as completely adhering to content and exposure, the study can be considered to have met fidelity.

In a perfect world, our participants would attend every session for the duration of the study. However, no matter how much we structure the protocol to account for the unexpected and unpredictability of "life", researchers need to be prepared for less than 100% adherence to the study protocol. Further, to be pragmatic, researchers need to let go of expecting the ideal dosage and instead consider what dosage is expected to effect a meaningful change in the participants. This is what we term "minimum" adherence. Minimum adherence is the absolute minimum intervention content and exposure needed to detect a clinically meaningful effect. Here, researchers must make a compromise between the ideal exposure and content, and that which is pragmatic and realistic. After all, creative arts therapists are working with humans whose complex lives mean that attendance and participation in all sessions (especially for long programs of several or more weeks) would perhaps be regarded as an overly optimistic expectation. The reality and the ideal is rarely the same. Participants may be too unwell to attend some sessions, they may have a competing commitment that cannot be rescheduled, they may have unexpected caring responsibilities, or they may just refuse to attend at times.

> *Case Study. Determining Minimum Adherence.* In our HOMESIDE study (Baker, Tamplin, et al., 2019; Baker et al., 2022) that compared a trained carer delivered music intervention program with a reading program and standard care, we proposed that a large effect in our main outcome measure would be observable following 5 × 30-minute music sharing experiences each week, for 12 weeks. This "dosage" for what of a better word, was considered the "ideal". However any change in wellbeing that can be directly modified by our planned intervention, we considered a good enough outcome. We anticipated that to detect any effect, the minimum adherence would be for careers to implement the music intervention programs at least 2 × 30-minutes per week, for at least 30 minutes in total per week, for 12 weeks. Any participant that averaged above this was considered to have met minimum adherence, and those below had not met minimum adherence.

Assessment of Intervention Components

Assessment of intervention components refers to the extent to which necessary (prescribed) elements within the intervention under examination are present, while excluding those that may "influence" the ability to confirm that it is the intervention and not some other factor that leads to the improved health outcome. Part of this process involves defining what are the unique features of the creative arts therapy approaches that are essential. In other words, without these components, the intervention would not have its "intended effect" (Carrol et al., 2007). However, the task of identifying the essential components of an intervention is complex. I will use a very concrete example—of the Bonny Method of Guided Imagery and Music (BM-GIM)—to illustrate this. One must first identify what components are *unique* and essential to an intervention. In the case of BM-GIM, it is unique and essential to use of all stages of prelude, induction, music program with accompanying imagery and guiding, mandala, discussion, and processing. These music programs for example have been previously described and tested for therapeutic use according to a range of musical and therapeutic considerations (Honig & McKinney, 2021). Second, identification of components that are essential to the intervention but not unique to it. For BM-GIM, this would include a verbal processing and reflection, which is also a core component for some psychotherapy and other creative arts therapies' approaches. The third element is that there are components of the intervention that are compatible to the intervention neither necessary nor unique (Nezu & Nezu, 2007). For BM-GIM, this could include selection of other music beyond the specific programs, curating different sequences of music selections rather than the suggested sequence, music listening without guided discussion, and discussion without music listening. And finally, there are components that are proscribed. For BM-GIM this would other methods such as improvisation, song writing and singing.

In identifying what components are unique but essential, essential but not unique, compatible, and proscribed, should inform the development of the intervention protocol, and therefore underpin the development of the fidelity measurement tool. However, this is not a straightforward a task. Further, it might not just be the individual components within an intervention that may impact the outcomes, but their combination and interactions. Using art therapy to illustrate, in a single-session art therapy program, the aim was for university students to visually explore a problem they were experiencing and how their world/life would look if the problem was resolved (Wilson, 2021). Within the intervention, participants selected images and used drawing to depict their view of the problem and life without the problem (unique and essential to the intervention) and experienced a verbal reflection (essential but not unique). Either one of these components could lead to positive outcomes, but it is their combination and interaction that is theorised to lead to the largest effect.

> *Case Example. Identifying Essential Components in International Trials Where Therapy Orientation Seems Incompatible.* Identifying the essential components has additional benefits when needing to adapt to different contexts. Our HOMESIDE RCT (Baker, Bloska, et al., 2019), where we implemented a family caregiver training program (indirect therapy, McDermott et al., 2018) was implemented in 5 countries—Australia, Norway, Germany, the United Kingdom, and Poland. Each of these countries have different music therapy traditions. The German tradition was strongly influenced by psychoanalytical approaches, the United Kingdom embeds psychodynamic thinking in their practice, while the Norwegian tradition more influenced by salutogenesis and humanistic traditions. In contrast, Polish and Australian practices are more eclectic, drawing on multiple orientations including practices neurologic music therapy, to meet different therapeutic needs. At face value, these traditions seem incompatible, therefore, one may question "how does a team of researchers with such diversity, arrive at an intervention protocol that includes essential and unique components, essential but not unique components, compatible but neither necessary or unique components, and proscribed components?". Such differences in music therapy traditions called for careful consideration.
>
> To navigate this challenge, researchers from each country met to discuss and arrive at a consensus based on experience and a review of research. While certain components of the intervention (i.e. specific activities) were agreed upon as essential to the intervention, the intervention protocol was developed in such a way as to allow for local variations in the delivery of them. Table 8.1 outlines the fidelity checklist items for the first music intervention carer training session. The items check for unique and essential content-related features of the intervention (explanations and demonstrations of activities) as well as delivery-related items such as more general therapeutic approaches that we agreed were essential, compatible, and common to each of the local traditions. For example, Item 1 under the category "General" states that "the interventionist is encouraging, supportive, and empathic throughout the training session". While each country may have a slightly different orientation in the way they implement this, we came to an agreement that despite the differences, it was compatible and therefore acceptable.

Table 8.1 Music intervention caregiver training fidelity checklist—training session 1

	Yes/no	Comments
Explanation		
1. Intention for intervention including a rationale and explanation of theory behind music use		
2. Commitment (sessions per week and time)		
3. Introduces all activities		
4. Explains all sections of the diary		
Activity 1. Singing familiar songs		
1. Interventionist assists caregiver to select culturally appropriate music/songs		
2. Interventionist assists caregiver to engage care recipient in song selection as needed		
3. Interventionist supports caregiver to engage their care recipient to sing familiar/preferred songs		
Activity 2. Movement/dancing to music		
1. Interventionist models either spontaneous OR directed movement to music for the caregiver		
2. Spontaneous movement: Interventionist models movement to music and/or responds to/mirrors participants' (care recipient and caregiver) spontaneous movements to music		
3. Directed movement: Interventionist models specific movements to music (e.g. dances associated with music/songs, specific exercises for head/neck, torso, arms, legs)		
4. Interventionist ensures that movements are appropriate for participants' physical abilities, interests, and attention span		
5. Interventionist assists dyad to select songs with upbeat tempo that are in keeping with participants' musical preferences and physical abilities		
Activity 3. Making music (optional)		
1. Interventionist explains how to use instrument/s available in participant homes (or how to use household items to create music)		
2. Interventionist models how to play along with recorded music and engage care recipient rhythmically		
Activity 4. Listening to Music (Relaxation)		
1. Interventionist explains and models breathing techniques to evoke a relaxed state		
2. Interventionist assists dyad to select songs with slow/relaxing tempo that are in keeping with participants' musical preferences		

(continued)

Table 8.1 (continued)

	Yes/no	Comments
3. Interventionist explains and models use of voice to evoke a relaxed state		
General		
1. The interventionist is encouraging, supportive and empathic throughout the training session (providing supportive feedback, tailoring approach to needs of the dyad)		
2. Interventionist encourages caregiver to engage care recipient through using eye contact, facial expression/s and gesture/s to encourage a response		
3. Interventionist encourages caregiver to mirror or reflect care recipients' spontaneous verbal and non-verbal responses (e.g. singing, vocalising, moving)		
4. Interventionist supports caregiver to engage care recipient in discussion related to selected songs and activities		

Caregiver—the person caring for their family member with dementia; Care recipient—the person living with dementia

The question remains however, as to how we identify and determine what the essential components in the creative arts therapies are when the intervention and therapy processes are highly complex? As mentioned earlier, reviewing the literature is one method of determining what the components essential to the intervention. Some common components of the creative arts therapies have been identified in a recent systematic review (De Witte et al., 2021). The review found there were several common factors shared with psychotherapy interventions (for example empathy, insight, expressive attunement). The review also identified joint factors common in at least two creative arts therapies (for example, embodiment, artistic agency), and specific factors (for example visual narrative, body awareness, doubling, musical attunement) which are only components of a single creative arts therapy discipline. But there is an even more systematic method of identifying the core components of an intervention—a component network meta-analysis. This specific form of meta-analysis will enable multiple interacting components of the intervention to be identified and defined (Rücker et al., 2020).

STRATEGIES TO SAFEGUARD THE QUALITY OF INTERVENTION DELIVERY

Once the intervention components and dose have been decided, the next task of the researcher is to establish processes that will lead to high-quality intervention implementation. Unlike drug studies, the experience, quality, and competence of the creative arts therapist to deliver the intervention can be a deciding factor in whether the intervention is highly effective, somewhat effective, ineffective, or potentially harmful. A well-developed and theoretically sound intervention protocol can still fail to be effective if not implemented to a high standard. In other words, the "quality of delivery is a potential moderator of the relationship between an intervention and the fidelity with which it is implemented" (Carroll et al., 2007). Conversely, an excellent and experienced clinician may be ineffective in delivering the planned intervention if there are not processes in place to monitor and ensure they implement as intended (Feely et al., p. 142).

With all this in mind, it is important to note that no studies exist in the creative arts therapies, nor in the evaluation of complex interventions more generally, that explore the relationship between implementation quality and the outcome. Further, while theoretically plausible, a search of the literature found that to date, there is not yet any research to confirm or disconfirm that implementing strategies to safeguard intervention quality has any impact on the degree of implementation fidelity.

There are several strategies that can be applied to increase the likelihood that the intervention implemented will be of a high standard and delivered according to the protocol. In short, these involve recruitment of excellent clinicians and the provision of extensive training, well-developed intervention materials, regular and ongoing supervision, and ongoing monitoring.

Creative Arts Therapist Competence and Training

In my 30+ years as a clinician and then researcher, I have engaged with many colleagues who employ creative arts therapy students or recent graduates to implement the interventions in their clinical trials. Reasons for this include availability (they have often not yet secured full-time, ongoing employment), and cost (students and newly graduated clinicians are "cheaper" to hire than more experienced clinicians). I would argue that hiring a more experienced clinician is always advisable, even if it, at face value, appears to be a greater strain on your research budget. From my perspective, experienced clinicians are more likely to be more effective (providing they follow the intervention protocol), thereby increasing the potential for the research to arrive at a significant outcome and with larger effect sizes. A big but not yet tested assumption, but a likely one. If spending a fraction more of you budget to employ more experienced clinicians over novices becomes the difference between achieving a large and smal effect, then it is an excellent financial investment.

All clinicians involved in a clinical trial will need to be trained in all aspects of the intervention implementation. Firstly, it is helpful to create position descriptions of the clinicians' role within the trial so they are clear about the requirements, experience, and proposed tasks. Ensure that when recruiting clinicians, that they are a good fit in terms of therapy orientation, experience with the specific population, and acceptance of the intervention approach. For example, a drama therapist practicing within a psychoanalytical orientation may find an intervention that involves cognitive reframing, inappropriate and may subsequently have difficulty authentically delivering the intervention described in the protocol.

Second, develop the intervention manual and training program, considering the content, sequence of content, and whether any practical/experiential components are needed. It is important to ensure that the training plan is driven by the protocol with special attention given to the theoretical underpinnings of the intervention and the necessary skills and requirements needed for effective treatment delivery (Borrelli, 2011). Further, training should focus on developing meta-competence so that interventionists understand the rationale behind the components. This will help them to implement the treatment components more authentically. Part of the discussions should focus on the proscribed elements of the intervention and the elements that might lead to treatment contamination.

The training should ensure all aspects around intervention implementation are outlined right from the outset. This includes important aspects such as how to set up the therapy room, materials used, documentation to complete, and closure of each session. Role plays and experiential components may be an integral component of the interventionist training program (Baker, Bloska, et al., 2019; Baker, Tamplin, et al., 2019). At the end of the training program, assessing the knowledge and skills of each interventionist is important so that the research team can be confident of their ability to implement the intervention as intended. If there are gaps in knowledge and skill identified, further training may be necessary. Possible items relevant and adapted from our MIDDEL (Baker, Tamplin, et al., 2019) and HOMESIDE (Baker, Bloska, et al., 2019) training questionnaires include:

1. What are the most effective ways of determining the music/art/dance/drama experiences and preferences of the participants?
2. Which research team members need to be masked to condition?
3. What are the three principle/theoretical (creative arts therapy specific) components that should be embedded in the session protocol?
4. What are the main sections of the session format?
5. What therapy techniques can you use to support participants' responses?
6. How would you go about encouraging interaction between participants?
7. What kinds of dialogue would you use to support (e.g. reminiscence, cognitive reframing, etc.)?
8. What would you do if a participant was not engaging with (the activity/therapy. etc.)?

9. How might you engage someone who is presenting as (e.g. apathetic, anxious, angry)?
10. What would you do if a participant became (e.g. agitated/aggressive, disruptive)?
11. What documentation needs to be recorded before the leaving the site?
12. Who should you contact from the research team if you are having issues with compliance from the site?
13. What do you do when a staff member from the site interrupts your therapy group?
14. Why is reviewing your video footage and completing a self-assessment important?

Intervention Supervision and Monitoring

While training creative arts therapists to implement the intervention according to the protocol is an integral component of the project plan, training is not a guarantee that interventionists will deliver as intended. Ongoing monitoring of the implementation is needed to safeguard against intervention drift (Borrelli, 2011). Drift is a concept that refers to a tendency for interventionists to gradually (and usually unknowingly) deviate from the intervention protocol. These may initially be subtle drifts, but over time these drifts may lead to an intervention consistently missing prescribed elements or other elements creeping into the sessions that were never intended. In some cases, these could be proscribed elements.

Supervision and monitoring may also be needed to assist some members of the team to negotiate an internal tension between their instinctual therapeutic responses to support client's immediate and ever-changing needs, with that of being a member of the research team required to adhere to a protocol. While ethical practice should always be at the forefront of the interventionists' minds and should never adhere to a protocol where there is a risk of causing harm, they also need to be mindful to keep the therapy sessions implemented as close to the protocol as possible and avoid unnecessary drift. This is particularly important when two interventions in a trial are similar (was was the case in MIDDEL when both interventions were music-based and could theoretically even contain the same choices in repertoire), and the research is focusing on identifying the impact of these nuanced differences on a specific health outcome. This is known as treatment differentiation and is described later in this chapter.

Ongoing monitoring can take the form of interventionists recording (or reviewing video footage) of their sessions immediately after implementing them, and cross checking these with the protocol. Checklists such as that presented in Table 8.1 provide a frame for interventionists to assess and reflect on their performance and be conscious to make adjustment in subsequent sessions as necessary. Similarly, it is important for other designated members of the research team to regularly review the interventionists' treatment implementation so that they can identify when drift begins to occur and correct it quickly.

Professional supervision can also be helpful to ensure interventionists do not drift from the protocol. During professional supervision, the supervisor together with the interventionist review video footage of sessions and discussing the general implementation of the intervention. Again, any deviations away from the intended protocol, can be quickly corrected. These sessions can also be used to improve the delivery of interventions in the same way that professional supervision supports creative arts therapy practitioners. This process becomes especially important in multi-site and international trials where it is essential that intervention implementation is adequately "comparable" across sites. Group supervision can assist in ensuring there are no treatment-by-site interactions (Borrelli, 2011). Choosing appropriately experienced clinicians who also understand the importance of protocol adherence, to provide the supervision is important.

In our MIDDEL (Baker, Tamplin, et al., 2019) (fidelity study) study, our supervision of interventionists uncovered that some interventionists are open and committed to strictly adhering to the protocol, while others tended to drift regularly. Such close monitoring can at times lead to tension between the therapists and the research team, but in my experience, sensitively communicating the need for strict adherence is usually received well.

Methods of Monitoring Adherence and Exposure

The measurement of adherence is predicated on the assumption that the specified content of an intervention can be measured and quantified (Ginsburg et al., 2021). Measurements will enable the research team to assess the extent to which the content of the intervention has been satisfactorily implemented, how frequently, and for how long. However, sometimes adherence may be met even when not all the components of the intervention were delivered (Ginsburg et al., 2021). For example, in the aforementioned example of HOMESIDE (Table 8.1), there were 19 assessable items once the items for the optional activity were excluded. After some discussion, the research team agreed that fidelity was met when 14 of the 19 assessable items were present. We then engaged independent reviewers who were not members of the research team to review video recordings of the sessions. We assert that such independent assessments minimise potential biased scoring and thus improves the research integrity of the trial.

Measuring "dose" is also a component of adherence that should be assessed for each participant. One might assume that if participants received what would be a low "dose" of their therapy program (for example attending very few sessions) that the effects would be lower than for other participants. This assumption is controversial and debatable as there is still a lot of "unknowns" about optimal dose. For example, in our MIDDEL study of residents with dementia in residential aged care homes, a participant was considered to have "attended" a 45-minute session so long as they were present for at least half of the session (23 minutes). This was based on the likelihood that many residents over the course of a 6-month program would have sessions where they were only there for part of the session due to reasons such as being brought to the session late, needing to leave for medical appointments or personal hygiene issues, etc. But this notion of attending and being present are not one and the same thing. We discussed at length how some participant may only be there for 15 minutes but if fully "present" for those 15 minutes may have had a greater therapeutic benefit than the resident who attended the whole 45 minutes but appeared asleep and with eyes closed for the entire session. Nevertheless, it's a randomised controlled trial and needs rules, so after much debate made the decision that attendance meant they were in attendance for at least 23 minutes. In the main outcome paper, we reported the percentage of participants who attended the minimum number of sessions and therefore met minimum adherence (Baker et al., 2022).

Dose when used in certain analyses can be used to determine either a "threshold effect" (where an effect does not occur until a certain dose has been reached, for example, at least 60% of full dose) or a "linear dose-response relationship" (the scenario where there are additional benefits for every increase in dose [sessions]) (Feely et al., 2018). Dose-adherence can also be explored at the "component" level. In this scenario, it may be that a particular component of the intervention—within a session or a specific session—is critical to consider the participant adhered sufficiently well to be considered in the per-protocol analyses. To illustrate, in our MAPS project (Music, psychology and social connects), an 8-session online group therapy program which combined psychology with music therapy was designed to promote wellbeing in couples where one partner had young onset dementia (Loi et al., 2022). There were seven topics covered, a different one each week, plus the introductory session. In week 5, there was a session that focused on exploring collaboration and communication between the couple. One of the outcome measures of the project, was the quality of caregiver-partner relationship as perceived by the carer, a commonly used measure (Spruytte et al., 2002). It is possible, that if a couple "missed" this session, that they may not demonstrate as much improvement (if any) when compared with participants who had attended this session.

Borrelli (2011) outlined the pros and cons of the two main methods of assessing treatment fidelity. The first is the review of audiotaped or video-recorded sessions. Where budget allows[2] and to strengthen the integrity of the data, this review is not usually undertaken by the clinician implementing the intervention, but an objective reviewer, and preferably someone independent of the trial with no conflict of interest. The reviewer can then compare the delivered intervention with the manualised version.

More general monitoring can also occur during professional supervision sessions led by the researcher in charge of intervention implementation. The supervisor will review sessions together with the therapist implementing the creative arts therapy interventions (or in some cases with the whole team of interventionists) to check and then correct any drift. The added advantage of this process is that the supervisor can

---

[2] Note that here I infer that this is best practice hence the caveat of "where budget allows" as I acknowledge here that best practice does cost money and many trials may have to sacrifice such best practice to make their budgets stretch further. For example, it may be a tradeoff between using funding resources to extend the trial to reach the target sample or reserving budget to fund an independent person to review the sessions to assess fidelity.

reinforce the importance of including the essential intervention components as well as creating opportunities for better standardisation of the intervention within and between interventionists. Another advantage to this approach is that it promotes accountability—that is, the interventionists are expected to provide high-quality interventions that meet protocol requirements, and the addition of regular checking means they are accountable, and therefore even more likely, to be faithful in their implementation.

The limitation of this method is that it can be obtrusive for participants and potentially impact their participation if they are aware that they are being audio or video recorded. Self-consciousness and anxiety may be experienced thereby impacting the potential benefits of the intervention and therefore the target outcome. Further, it may impact clinicians' sense of "ease" when delivering the intervention, as they may experience this as being "under the microscope". Here, it is helpful if the supervisor in charge of reviewing the intervention footage reinforces the reason for the review—it's for content and fidelity to the intention of the intervention, not a review of their quality of practice as such. Reinforcing that the reason they have been chosen as an interventionist for the trial is because of their expertise and high standard of practice.

The second approach to monitoring adherence and prevention of drift is to use intervention self-report checklists. After each session is delivered, interventionists may be required to immediately complete a checklist to record their actions and provide explanations for any deviations from the proposed plan. Completing this checklist serves as a prompt to remind to them about the critical components of the intervention. Adherence may improve if they recognise that after each session provided, they must create a report on whether each component is delivered, and if not, to provide an explanation for why. When used as a fidelity checklist, this approach is valuable in supplementing more direct methods of assessment but can be subject to bias as they may rate themselves as being more adherent than the reality. The final approach to monitor adherence is through participant self-report. Here, study participants are asked to check off what was included in the therapy sessions. It can also offer opportunities for assessing nonspecific process issues such as feeling listened to versus rushed, feeling understood versus uncomfortable, or feeling respected versus criticised (Borrelli, 2011, p. S54).

Treatment Receipt

Participant responsiveness refers to the extent whereby participants are actively engaged, enthusiastic, interactive, and receptive to the intervention (Feely et al., 2018). It is well understood across the creative arts therapies that participants are active in their efforts towards better health, and this active role involves them engaging fully with, understanding, and acquiring intervention-related skills. This is known as treatment receipt. A disengaged participant who does not understand the relevance and utility is unlikely to experience the same response to the intervention when compared with an engaged participant (Carrol et al., 2007).

Treatment receipt falls into four related categories, all of which are rarely reported in research studies (Borrelli et al., 2005; Rixon et al., 2016). The first concerns the provisions of processes to determine whether the participants understand the purpose or content of an intervention they are engaged in. For example, does the participant understand that the purpose behind an art engagement experience is to express thoughts and feelings that are difficult to access and transform them concrete into something concrete. The second category is the incorporation of pre-planned strategies to improve participants' understanding of the intervention. An example of this might be to highlight to a participant when a certain action, verbalisation, or artistic expression occurs and then offer feedback as to how the intervention stimulated that response. The third category relates to the assessment of participants' abilities to perform/engage with the tasks and experiences that are offered during the therapy program. An example of this from within our HOMESIDE study is where we are guiding family carers of people with dementia to use music to support care (Baker, Bloska, et al., 2019). Within the session, we can observe how much they have learned and are able to apply the skills within the training session and provide feedback to ensure they understand. If carers are to implement sessions following our training program, we need to feel confident that they understand the content and can perform the required tasks. The final category of treatment receipt relates to strategies embedded in the trial to improve participants' performance of intervention skills. Building on the previous example within HOMESIDE, we conducted fortnightly phone calls during participants' intervention period so that we could discuss any challenges they had in using the skills they had been taught and further refining these skills.

Table 8.2 outlines examples of where creative arts therapists could assess treatment receipt.

Table 8.2 Treatment receipt examples in creative arts therapy research

Treatment receipt category	Creative arts therapy example	Treatment receipt measurement purpose
Intervention components received or completed	Participant offered a specific art activity to engage in, and participant completes task	Assessing of intervention understanding
Problem areas discussed	Drama therapist/participants discuss barriers to participant	Strategies to improve performance of intervention skills
Treatment satisfaction	Participant completes a session evaluation form after each dance/movement session	Assessing of intervention understanding
Engagement (level of participation, involvement, enjoyment, or communication)	Drama therapist assesses the extent to which participants involved themselves in the dramatic experience	Assessing of intervention understanding
Attendance[a]	Monitoring attendance of participants at therapeutic choir program	Assessing of intervention understanding
Acceptability	Participants ongoing reporting of relevance/capacity/willingness to participate in dance/movement sessions to	Assessing of intervention understanding
In-session trialling of new learning	Observation of participant experimenting with new art materials	Assessing abilities to perform the intervention skills
Use of materials (homework completed)	Participants in art therapy complete reflective diary during program	Assessing of intervention understanding
Telephone contacts during intervention period	Regular phone calls to discuss implementation of music intervention, discuss problems, and refine skills	Strategies to improve performance of intervention skills
Reaction/feedback on intervention	Drama therapist offers insights into participant's dramatic expression	Strategies to improve performance of intervention skills

[a]Attendance can be an indicator of how satisfied/engaged/relevant an intervention is to the participants as well as being an indicator of adherence (see earlier discussion)

Treatment Differentiation

Treatment differentiation is a term used to describe the degree to which two or more of the study arms within a trial differ according to critical dimensions (Borrelli, 2011). While many creative arts therapies are comparing a creative art therapy with either standard care and/or another non-arts-based therapies (e.g. psychotherapy), there is increasing interest in comparing creative arts therapies against an intervention that involves artistic engagement but not delivered by a credentialed therapist. In such cases, treatment differentiation is essential so that the interventions remain conceptually and practically distinct. This becomes even more critical when the same therapist may provide differing treatment interventions. Processes such as clear manuals with operationalised definitions linked to theory and ongoing monitoring of the intervention delivery will assist in ensuring that two or more therapies are distinguishable. As an illustration of this, our study compared small group music therapy delivered by a credentialed music therapist, with group singing delivered by a community musician MIDDEL (Baker, Tamplin, et al., 2019). The theoretical basis for these two interventions guided the design of the protocol and assisted in identifying the distinguishable elements of the two. The group music therapy interventions emphasised individualised in-the-moment musical responding to participants' responses with the aim of regulating emotions. It was informed by personhood and psychosocial models of music in dementia. Conversely, the mechanisms underpinning the choir singing intervention were more focused on cognitive stimulation and social interaction (Gold et al., 2019). In this study, it was important to monitor the interventions being delivered in different treatment arms so that the distinction between the two interventions was maintained throughout the study.

Treatment Enactment

Treatment enactment involves the assessment, monitoring, and improvement of the abilities of participants to translate and integrate their skills, strategies, and learning derived from their therapies into their everyday life (Borrelli, 2011). Where possible, it focuses on assessing, monitoring, and improving the appropriateness and timing of the use of these skills relevant to the context (Bellg et al., 2004). While treatment delivery aims to influence health and treatment receipt concerns assessing whether skills are learned within sessions, enactment goes beyond both of these to determine whether they can be applied outside of the clinical/research setting.

Several strategies can be adopted to assess enactment. Most common are direct observation or self-report. HOMESIDE illustrates both of these. To recap, the music therapist provides three carer training sessions, the first after baseline, then a second, and third session three and six weeks later. The idea behind these sessions is threefold—(1) to provide support and encouragement so that the intervention will be implemented (adherence), (2) to provide extension training sessions (treatment receipt), and (3) to observe how the carer applies the skills learned in earlier training sessions in the home context (observed treatment enactment). Self-report of enactment is also captured through fortnightly phone calls with the interventionists and through recorded diary entries of music use. Here, the carers report what, where, when, how, why, and with what effect they used music to support the care of their loved one. This provides insight into how they can use the learned skills in context.

Conclusion

Evaluation of intervention fidelity is a crucial process for safeguarding research integrity. Without it, the outcomes of the study may be questioned. Establishing good fidelity processes is also helpful in that it can improve intervention quality. It is important to plan for fidelity processes early in the study design, and to consider the resources needed to engage in it fully. The aspects of fidelity described in this chapter are not intended to be a rigid set of rules, but more to stimulate thoughts and reflections on how to best design fidelity processes in creative arts therapies trials. Actively embedding rigorous fidelity checks will raise the quality of the research, and thus lead to more policy-changing opportunities.

References

Baker, F. A., Bloska, J., Stensæth, K., Wosch, T., Bukowska, A., Braat, S., Sousa, T., Tamplin, J., Clark, I. N., Lee, Y.-E. C., Clarke, P., Lautenschlager, N., & Odell-Miller, H. (2019). HOMESIDE: A home-based family caregiver-delivered music intervention for people living with dementia: Protocol of a randomised controlled trial. *British Medical Journal Open*. https://doi.org/10.1136/bmjopen-2019-031332

Baker, F. A., Lee, Y.-E. C., Sousa, T. V., Stretton-Smith, P. A., Tamplin, J., Sveinsdottir, V., Geretsegger, M., Wake, J. D., Assmus, J., & Christian Gold, C. (2022). Clinical effectiveness of Music Interventions for Dementia and Depression in Elderly care (MIDDEL) in the Australian cohort: pragmatic cluster-randomised controlled trial. *The Lancet Healthy Longevity, 3*(3), e153–e165. https://doi.org/10.1016/S2666-7568(22)00027-7

Baker, F. A., Tamplin, J., Clark, I., Lee, Y.-E. C., Geretsegger, M., & Gold, C. (2019). Treatment fidelity in a music therapy multi-site cluster randomized control trial for people living with dementia: The MIDDEL project. *Journal of Music Therapy*. https://doi.org/10.1093/jmt/thy023

Bellg, A. J., Borrelli, B., Resnick, B., Hecht, J., Minicucci, D. S., Ory, M., Ogedegbe, G., Orwig, D., Ernst, D., Czajkowski, S., & Treatment Fidelity Workgroup of the NIH Behavior Change Consortium. (2004). Enhancing treatment fidelity in health behavior change studies: Best practices and recommendations from the NIH Behavior Change Consortium. *Health Psychology, 23*, 443–451. https://doi.org/10.1037/0278-6133.23.5.443

Borrelli, B. (2011). The assessment, monitoring, and enhancement of treatment fidelity in public health clinical trials. *Journal of Public Health Dentistry, 71*(Supp/1), S52–S63. Apologies its a sole authored publication.

Borrelli, B., Sepinwall, D., Ernst, D., Bellg, A. J., Czajkowski, S., Breger, R., DeFrancesco, C., Levesque, C., Sharp, D. L., Ogedegbe, G., Resnick, B., & Orwig, D. (2005). A new tool to assess treatment fidelity and evaluation of treatment fidelity across 10 years health behavior research. *Journal of Consulting and Clinical Psychology, 73*, 852–860. https://doi.org/10.1037/0022-006X.73.5.852

Carroll, C., Patterson, M., Wood, S., Booth, A., Rick, J., & Balain, S. (2007). A conceptual framework for implementation fidelity. *Implementation Science, 2*, 40–48. https://doi.org/10.1186/1748-5908-2-40

Chan, C. K. P., Lo, T. L. T., Wan, A. H. Y., Leung, P. P. Y., Pang, M. Y. C., & Ho, R. T. H. (2021). A randomised controlled trial of expressive arts-based intervention for young stroke survivors. *BMC Complementary Medicine and Therapies, 21*(1), 7. https://doi.org/10.1186/s12906-020-03161-6

De Witte, M., Orkibi, H., Zarate, R., Karkou, V., Sanjani, N., Malhotra, B., Ho, R. T. H., Kaimal, G., Baker, F. A., & Koch, S. C. (2021). Identifying mechanisms of change for psychological health outcomes in the creative arts therapies. A scoping review. *Frontiers in Psychology, 12*, 678397. Published online 15 July 2021. https://doi.org/10.3389/fpsyg.2021.678397

Dusenbury, L., Brannigan, R., Falco, M., & Hansen, W. (2003). A review of research on fidelity of implementation: Implications for drug abuse prevention in school settings. *Health Education Research, 18*, 237–256.

Feely, M., Seay, K. D., Lanier, P., Auslander, W., & Kohl, P. L. (2018). Measuring fidelity in research studies: A field guide to developing a comprehensive fidelity measurement system. *Child & Adolescent Social Work Journal, 35*(2), 139–152. https://doi.org/10.1007/s10560-017-0512-6

Feniger-Schaal, R., & Orkibi, H. (2020). Integrative systematic review of drama therapy intervention research. *Psychology of Aesthetics Creativity and the Arts, 14*(1), 68–80. https://doi.org/10.1037/aca0000257

Fong, Z. H., Tan, S. H., Mahendran, R., Kua, E. H., & Chee, T. T. (2021). Arts-based interventions to improve cognition in older persons with mild cognitive impairment: A systematic review of randomized controlled trials. *Aging & Mental Health, 25*(9), 1605–1617.

Ginsburg, L. R., Hoben, M., Easterbrook, A., Anderson, R. A., Estabrooks, C. A., & Norton, P. G. (2021). Fidelity is not easy! Challenges and guidelines for assessing fidelity in complex interventions. *Trials, 22*(1). https://doi.org/10.1186/s13063-021-05322-5

Gold, C., Eickholt, J., Assmus, J., Stige, B., Wake, J. D., Baker, F. A., ... Geretsegger, M. (2019). Music Interventions for Dementia and Depression in Elderly care (MIDDEL): Protocol and statistical analysis plan for a multi-national cluster-randomised trial. *BMJ Open, 9*(3), 14. https://doi.org/10.1136/bmjopen-2018-023436

Honig, T. J., & McKinney, C. H. (2021). Monitoring variation to Guided Imagery and Music (GIM): Development of the GIM Treatment Fidelity Instrument. *Nordic Journal of Music Therapy, 30*(5), 440–459. https://doi.org/10.1080/08098131.2021.1888781

Loi, S. M., Flynn, L., Cadwallader, C., Stretton-Smith, P., Bryant, C., & Baker, F. A. (2022). Music and psychology and social connections program: Protocol for a novel intervention for dyads affected by younger-onset dementia. *Brain Sciences, 12*(4), 503. https://doi.org/10.3390/brainsci12040503

McDermott, O., Ridder, H. M. O., Stige, B., Ray, K., Wosch, T., & Baker, F. A. (2018). Indirect music therapy practice and skill-sharing for dementia care. *Journal of Music Therapy.* https://doi.org/10.1093/jmt/thy012

Mihalic, S. (2004). The importance of implementation fidelity. *Emotional & Behavioral Disorders in Youth, 4*, 99–105.

Moncher, F. J., & Prinz, F. J. (1991). Treatment fidelity in outcome studies. *Clinical Psychology Review, 11*, 247–266. https://doi.org/10.1016/0272-7358(91)90103-2

Nezu, A. M., & Nezu, C. M. (2007). Ensuring treatment integrity. In A. M. Nezu & C. M. Nezu (Eds.), Evidence-based outcome research: A practical guide to conducting randomized controlled trials for psychosocial interventions (pp. 499–534). Oxford University Press, Incorporated, 2007.

Proctor, E., Silmere, H., Raghavan, R., Hovmand, P., Aarons, G., Bunger, A., Griffey, R., & Hensley, M. (2011). Outcomes for implementation research: Conceptual distinctions, measurement challenges, and research agenda. *Administration and Policy in Mental Health and Mental Health Services Research, 38*(2), 65–76.

Rixon, L., Baron, J., McGale, N., Lorencatto, F., Francis, J., & Davies, A. (2016). Methods used to address fidelity of receipt in health intervention research: A citation analysis and systematic review. *BMC Health Service Research, 16,* 663. https://doi.org/10.1186/s12913-016-1904-6

Robb, S. L., Burns, D. S., & Carpenter, J. S. (2011). Reporting guidelines for music-based interventions. *Journal of Health Psychology, 16*(2), 342–352. https://doi.org/10.1177/1359105310374781

Robb, S. L., Hanson-Abromeit, D., May, L., Hernandez-Ruiz, E., Allison, M., Beloat, A., Daugherty, S., Kurtz, R., Oyedele, O. O., Polasik, S., Rager, A., Rifkin, J., & Wolf, E. (2018). Reporting quality of music intervention research in healthcare: A systematic review. *Complementary Therapies in Medicine, 38,* 24–41. https://doi.org/10.1016/j.ctim.2018.02.008

Roen, K., Arai, L., Roberts, H., & Popay, J. (2006). Extending systematic reviews to include evidence on implementation: Methodological work on a review of community-based initiatives to prevent injuries. *Social Science and Medicine, 63,* 1060–1071.

Rücker, G., Petropoulou, M., & Schwarzer, G. (2020). Network meta-analysis of multicomponent interventions. *Biometrical Journal, 62*(3), 808–821. https://doi.org/10.1002/bimj.201800167. Epub 2019 April 25. PMID: 31021449; PMCID: PMC7217213.

Spruytte, N., Van Audenhove, C., Lammertyn, F., & Storms, G. (2002). The quality of the caregiving relationship in informal care for older adults with dementia and chronic psychiatric patients. *Psychology and Psychotherapy: Theory, Research and Practice, 75*(3), 295–311. https://doi.org/10.1348/147608302320365208

Suskin, G., & Al-Yagon, M. (2020). Culturally sensitive dance movement therapy for ultra-orthodox women: Group protocol targeting bodily and psychological self-perceptions. *The Arts in Psychotherapy, 71.*

Walton, H., Spector, A., Tombor, I., & Michie, S. (2017). Measures of fidelity of delivery of, and engagement with, complex, face-to-face health behaviour change interventions: A systematic review of measure quality. *British Journal of Health Psychology, 22*(4), 1–19. https://doi.org/10.1111/bjhp.12260

Wilson, E. (2021). Novel solutions to student problems: A phenomenological exploration of a single session approach to art therapy with creative arts university students. *Frontiers in Psychology, 11.* https://doi.org/10.3389/fpsyg.2020.600214

CHAPTER 9

Statistical Analysis Plan

What Is a Statistical Analysis Plan?

One of the many but serious threats to research integrity is the potential for research bias that may occur during the statistical analysis process. The Statistical Analysis Plan (SAP) is a key document for any clinical trial that contains detailed descriptions of statistical analyses to be conducted (Yuan et al., 2019). It contains details of the trial, including rationale for choice of statistical methods, plans for dealing with unexpected difficulties, and pre-specified direction on interpretation of the results. While the study protocol will always outline the statistical approaches to be employed in the trial, the SAP provides extensive, more technical, and detailed explanations of statistical approaches to be adopted (Yuan et al., 2019).

Why Does a Trial Need a Statistical Analysis Plan?

It is a given that statistical decisions made by the research team will influence the trial outcomes and therefore a transparent and trustworthy documented statistical plan is essential (Gamble et al., 2017). Not only will this plan improve trustworthiness of the outcomes, but it enables a third party to reproduce the outcomes if given the data set. Although I have yet to experience this, when the trustworthiness of the results is called into question by another researcher or journal editor, a good SAP plan will enable the third party to request access to the data and re-run the same statistical methods. Following the detailed protocol will ensure that the findings are replicated and therefore defendable.

Like all other components within a clinical trial, the statistical analysis should be planned, developed, and decided on by the team prior to finalising the data cleaning and then subsequent lockdown of the database. This process removes the temptation for researchers to "interrogate the data intensively and extensively" (DeMets et al., 2017) and to conduct multiple unplanned or post-hoc analyses to obtain maximum benefit from a data set (known as data dredging (Finfer & Bellomo, 2009). The more outcomes, subgroups, and variables tested, the greater the chance of a false-positive finding.[1] When there are multiple outcomes and relationships between outcomes of interest, the research team needs to decide which ones are of the most interest, with a clear decision about which outcome variable is the primary one. This will prevent researchers from selectively reporting results that "look interesting" or manipulating the reporting of data to only present those which support efficacy (Finfer & Bellomo, 2009). From there, the remaining outcomes should be specified and ordered in the degree of importance. Further, any subgroup analyses should be small and ranked and ordered according to their level of importance (DeMets et al., 2017).

Lastly, it is well recognised that there may be numerous statistical approaches to testing the effects of outcome measures. Different biostatisticians support different approaches and having sat on several discussions with teams of biostatisticians, it is fascinating (to a non-statistical expert) to witness the discussions and debate about the different options under consideration. To prevent researchers from the poor practice of running multiple tests and "shopping around" until they find a method that leads to the best results, pre-defining the statistical methods is important. Any methods that are likely to influence the outcomes such as secondary evaluations, sensitivity analyses and even how missing data is handled, should also be predefined (DeMets et al., 2017; Gamble et al., 2017). It is now an increasingly more common practice to make publicly available the statistical analysis plan prior to completing the study, and many research

---

[1] A false-positive occurs when the statistical analyses find a positive change because of the creative arts therapy intervention, when one does not actually exist. The more analyses that are run, the more likely based on probability, that a significant outcome will be detected.

groups publish their plans in peer reviewed journals. At the time of writing this book, our HOMESIDE team were in the final stages of drafting the SAP for publication ahead of database lockdown.

Developing a Statistical Analysis Plan

The SAP may be described within the study protocol (Chapter 2) and/or manual of procedures (Chapter 2), but more increasingly, it is a stand-alone document. The first version of the SAP is normally developed prior to enrolling the first study participant and should be approved by the trial statistician, the research team, and the Data Safety Monitoring Board (Chapter 3). Some ethics review boards may want to review the SAP prior to providing ethical approval. The trial statistician(s) usually author the SAP but the research team do have input into the contents and make critical decisions such as choice of primary and secondary outcomes, and in clinical interpretation of results. It is usual practice for the document to be under "strict version control" and every new version is electronic-date-stamped.

Gamble et al. (2017) undertook a Delphi study to develop guidelines for the content of the SAP. Their study identified 55 items that were important contents of the plan. They fell into six main categories: (1) administrative information, (2) a synopsis of the trial background, rationale, and objectives, (3) study methods, (4) general statistical conventions, (5) descriptions of the trial population, and (6) outcome definitions and analysis methods. Each of these are described in detail.

The first part of the SAP provides important administrative information and is often presented in a single cover page of the document. It begins with the title of the trial and includes the SAP often as a subtitle. It also includes the ever increasingly popular trial acronym—for example, in our projects, MIDDEL, MATCH, HOMESIDE, RemiSing, and MAPs. This section details the trial registration number, the statistical analysis plan version history, a justification for each SAP revision, and the timing of the revisions in relation to any interim analyses,[2] etc. Following this section,

---

[2] An interim analysis is an evaluation of current data from an ongoing trial. It focuses on the primary research question and outcomes and may influence the conduct of the trial including whether to modify the sample size, study design, early indication of success, or early termination. It may also be used to guide cost and resource allocation (Kumar & Chakraborty, 2016).

the names, affiliations, roles, and responsibilities of the SAP contributors are listed. Finally, the signatures of the person authoring the SAP, senior statistician and principal investigator are added.

The next section of the protocol provides relevant information about the background of the trial and a justification for its implementation. Clear descriptions of the specific objectives and hypotheses to be tested should be included which replicate what is detailed in the study protocol. The next section should include a brief description of the trial method, making sure that the text includes (a) trial design, (b) description of the interventions, (c) randomisation details including plans to stratify, (d) the sample size along with information about how the required sample size was determined, and finally, what hypothesis testing framework is being used (whether the trial tests for superiority, equivalency, or non-inferiority).[3] Included in this section are the plans (including timepoints) for performing any interim analyses and whether adjustments will be made because of the analyses. Further, guidance for stopping the trial prior to completion need to be detailed. The section should also include the timing of outcome assessments including the permissible "windows" for collecting data. For example, in our HOMESIDE trial, the window for assessment at all timepoints (21, 42, and 90 days) was ±7 days for all scheduled assessment dates (Baker et al., 2019). Anything data collected outside of this ±7 days window was considered a protocol violation. Soon after commencing the trial, it became apparent that this window was not pragmatic within the complex lives of people living in the community, and the pandemic increased the challenge in meeting this window. It was subsequently adjusted to ±14 days and this was published in the final SAP. What is considered an acceptable window will differ between studies dependent upon study design and expected rate of change. To contrast the HOMESIDE study example, our delirium study was based on 3 consecutive days of intervention. For each day, post-data collection needed to be completed within 30 minutes of a session completion (Golubovic et al., under review; study protocol registered).

The next section outlines the statistical principles that will underpin the analyses. Descriptions of confidence intervals and p-values are stated

---

[3] Superiority, equivalency, or non-inferiority trials are those that aim to test whether one intervention is superior to another intervention (superiority), that two treatments are not too different in their targeted effects (equivalency) or that the intervention undergoing testing is not worse than standard care (Lesaffre, 2008).

including the level of statistical significance expected, and descriptions and rationales for adjustments made for multiple comparisons (and how Type I error will be controlled[4]).

A detailed description of the adherence and protocol deviations is also needed. First, the SAP should describe how adherence is assessed and by whom. To illustrate, in our HOMESIDE study, we recommended that family carers engage the person with dementia in five 30-minute sessions of music engagement per week, for 12 weeks. This "dosage" figure was based on findings from prior research and informed by clinical practice as "ideal" to achieve the best therapeutic outcomes. Note that I used the word "ideal" here. In the case of HOMESIDE, we hypothesised that five weekly sessions would provide maximum benefit however in reality, we agreed that it was unlikely most of our study participants would be able to achieve this. So it became a question of what the "minimum" number of sessions would be to affect change. Again, based on prior research findings, we hypothesised that a minimum of two sessions per week totalling 30-minute sessions per week was likely to effect some change and was therefore considered our minimum adherence. To capture adherence, participants completed a diary throughout the trial, and they were contacted by members of the research team once per fortnight to check that the diaries were being completed. These processes were defined in the SAP.

In addition, this section also describes the study population. Contents detail eligibility criteria, recruitment approaches, as well as how screening will be reported to allow descriptions for how representative the included participant sample is in the main outcomes paper. Plans for how to deal with withdrawals/follow-ups, and the timing and reasons for these will be outlined, and finally details of how the baseline characteristics will be summarised are documented.

The final section of the SAP presents the analysis approach. It first describes the outcomes to be tested including the timing of primary and secondary endpoints, the measurement tools (and any data concerning reliability and validity), any approach to calculate or transform the measures to derive the outcome (e.g. changes from baseline, transformations on QoL measures into quality adjusted life years, etc.). Following this, the SAP details the methods used and how treatment effects will

---

[4] A Type I error occurs when the null hypothesis is rejected when its actually true.

be presented. Adjustment for covariates is detailed alongside methods used for checking assumptions. If methods are to be used when assumptions are not distributed, details of these need to be described. Planned sensitivity and/or subgroup analyses should also be included.

While good data management (Chapter 7) aims to reduce the amount of missing data, it is quite common in psychosocial intervention research studies to have missing data. Creative arts therapies research are not exempt from this likelihood either. Within the SAP plan, there needs to be explanations and justifications for how to treat missing data for each individual outcome measure. Treatment of missing data is discussed more fully later in this chapter with examples to illustrate the various approaches.

Importantly, the SAP needs to clearly specify how data on participant safety will be collected and reported. For example, it needs to articulate what event is classified as a serious adverse event compared with a mild adverse event. It also needs to articulate how that information is being collected to classify the event into its level of severity, expectedness, and causality.[5] In planning the SAP in HOMESIDE, we collected data from the two assessment timepoints (post-intervention and follow-up), as well as regularly sourced from the clinicians during the three music training sessions, and the fortnightly phone calls.

The final section of the SAP is to outline the various statistical software that is planned to be utilised in the analyses—for example SPSS, R, Minitab—and details of these and their versions should be noted. Any relevant references to important information such as nonstandard statistical methods and the data management plan should be included.

---

[5] Adverse events are those where there are changes in health and wellbeing that are considered inappropriate or undesirable. In the case of our MATCH, study which is involved in detecting and regulating agitation in people living with dementia using continuously adapted music, adverse event might be that on the day that music was used, the person with dementia had difficulty settling at night. A serious adverse event is characterised as a treatment reaction that is life-threatening or leads to death, hospitalisation, disability, etc. In the case of MATCH, if a person's level of agitation increased (as opposed to decreased) and it leads the person to stand up unexpectedly, fall, and break their neck of femur (hip), this would be regarded as a serious adverse event.

Statistical Analysis Plan for Observational Studies

While documenting and registering SAPs are almost business as usual now in randomised controlled trials, there is an increasing expectation that SAPs will also be developed and registered for observational studies (*The Lancet*, 2010). Just as is the case for randomised controlled trials, it can be argued that a predefined SAP can improve the quality and rigor of observational studies. Careful planning will lead to an avoidance of indiscriminate analyses, optimises statistical resources to analyse the most important questions, and facilitates transparency (Thomas & Peterson, 2012). As these studies are not randomised trials, some key information in a RCT SAP is not relevant in observational studies. Such items include randomisation, adherence, and protocol deviations. Those researchers who are undertaking observational studies are encouraged to review the SAP guidelines by Hiemstra et al. (2019) and Yuan et al. (2019).

Missing Data

As discussed in Chapter 7, good data management will enable the trial to have the best chance of collecting a high quality and complete data set. However, in my experience, it is rare to complete a moderate size, let alone a large size trial with a complete data set; missing data is a reality of implementing trials. It is how we deal with it that allows us to minimise its impact. The challenge of missing data is that it can reduce statistical power, can lead to biasing the estimation of parameters, can decrease the representativeness of the sample, and can introduce complexities in the statistical analysis process. Each of these may lead to threats to the validity of the study and the trustworthiness of its conclusions (Kang, 2013).

Within clinical research studies, there are three types of missing data—missing completely at random, missing at random, and missing not at random. *Missing completely at random* is understood as missing data that has no connection with the characteristics or responses of the participant being studied. In the creative arts therapies, these could take the form of questionnaires that went missing in the post, questionnaire responses captured electronically were not properly submitted, uploaded or saved, or data capturing equipment such as microphones or voice-capture equipment, EEG recordings, video recordings, failed to capture the data to be analysed. From a statistical analysis perspective, the loss of these forms of data is unbiased. Therefore, while it impacts the power of the study, the estimated parameters are not biased by the missing data (Kang, 2013).

The second type of missing data is *missing at random*. This type of missingness has to do with the participant but can be predicted from other information about the participant. One example could be that males are less likely to complete a survey about depression, and this has nothing to do with their level of depression (Mack et al., 2018). In other words, certain characteristics of participants that have nothing to do with the phenomenon under investigation, may lead to missing data. In our HOMESIDE study, data on adherence was collected by the family carers of people with dementia, via their completion of a specifically designed diary. While those carers who were life partners/spouses of the person with dementia were relatively consistent in completing the diary, those adult children who had competing work and child-caring responsibilities were more likely to have missing entries in the diary. This does not relate to the intervention, or the type of data being collected hence it is still regarded as missing at random.

Finally, *missing not at random* is data whereby the missingness is related to what is missing. Within creative arts clinical trials, this often relates to data capturing the emotional wellbeing of participants. Using the example of people with depression (in this case irrespective of gender), when trying to capture data on the impact of an intervention on depression, it is likely that those participants with severe depression are more likely to provide and complete the survey or refuse entirely to provide responses to the questions. Such missing data does introduce bias.

Approaches to Treat Missing Data

Several approaches can be used to treat missing data all of which need to be clearly described in the SAP and reported in any publication of the findings. While an in depth understanding of these is not required of a principal investigator—it's the specific domain of the biostatistical team—an overview and basic understanding of the different approaches as I provide here, can assist the principal investigator to understand how the research data is being treated.[6]

The most common approach is to omit an entire case (*case deletion*). This might be appropriate in studies with large sample sizes and where the study is adequately powered to detect differences with a reduced data set. In such studies, deleting a small number of cases will not have a detrimental impact on the outcomes. This may not be the case in studies with smaller sample sizes. Here, every participant's data counts. For every case deletion, there is a greater chance that power is not achieved and that an inconclusive finding will be reached.

The second approach is *pairwise deletion*. It is often the case that there may data missing in one variable but not others. This is particularly apparent in studies where there is data collected from multiple sources (staff, participants, family, etc.). For any number of reasons, data from one source may be missing. Data collected from staff report may be missing because they were too busy on the ward or were absent on the planned data collection day. Data from family may be missing because they failed to return the phone calls despite the research team's efforts to make repeated contact, or the study participants themselves (clients), may be unable to self-report due to health reasons or some other unexpected factor that occurred on the day of data collection. In such cases, the data from the remaining variables will be included in the analysis for that participant. In our HOMESIDE study, data was collected from the family carer and the person living with dementia. In some cases, the person living with dementia was not well enough to complete their self-report data (Quality of Life-Alzheimer's Disease), so this data was missing not at random and not used in the analyses, but all other data for that participant including the main outcome measure (Neuropsychiatric Inventory-Questionnaire) was included. *Pairwise deletion* is permissible in correlation, factor, quick cluster, and regression analyses. It is a less biased approach when data is missing at random or missing completely at random (Kang, 2013).

---

[6] While it may not be necessary to understand how the statistical team arrived at their choices for treating missing data—or analysing any data within the trial—it is important as a researcher to understand how missing data was captured, categorised, and addressed within the analyses as extent and type of missingness and procedures to treating missing data will impact the findings.

The third approach is *simple imputation* (Jakobsen et al., 2017). There are three types—mean substitution, last observed carried forward, worst observation carried forward. For *mean substitution*, the missing data is replaced with the whole sample's mean value for that variable. This approach allows researchers to utilise collected data to create a more complete data set (Kang, 2013). This approach can be used at the level of an individual item within an outcome measure (e.g. one item in a depression scale) or can be used for the measures total score. The larger the sample size, the more minor the impact of such an approach has on the findings.

The single imputation method of *last observation carried forward* addresses missing data at the participant rather than whole sample level. Here, a participant's missing score at a certain timepoint is replaced with their score on the same item/total measure score from the previous timepoint. This approach is used commonly in longitudinal/repeated measures studies. Using the MIDDEL study as an example (Baker et al., 2022), data was collected at four timepoints (baseline, mid-intervention, post-intervention, follow-up). As we had COVID-19-related interruptions to the study, some data was not able to be completed as we had no way to access the participants in the residential aged care home during lockdowns. Therefore, whole data sets for some participants were missing at the mid-intervention timepoint (not the primary timepoint). Their data at the mid-intervention timepoint was replaced by their baseline data. While this allows for a more complete data set to be analysed, the disadvantage of this approach is that it assumes the value of the outcome remains unchanged and should not be used as the main approach to treatment of missing data (Kang, 2013). Similar to the last observed carried forward approach is the *worst observation carried forward* approach replaces missing values with the participant's worse observed values.

Studies suggest that single imputation methods are based on several assumptions that have been viewed as unrealistic, introducing potential bias. Therefore, they should be used with caution (Jorgensen et al., 2014).

Multiple imputation is another approach to dealing with missing data. Here, missing data is replaced through a statistical modelling process that involves creating several different "plausible" imputed data sets and

> *Treatment of Missing Data in HOMESIDE trial.* "To describe the missing data, the frequency and percentage of participants with a missing value at baseline, 3-months post-randomisation and 6-months post-randomisation will be summarised for all study variables overall and by treatment arm for the intention-to-treat population. Where available, reasons for the missingness will be tabulated. In addition, baseline and demographic characteristics will be summarised overall and for those with and without a missing value at baseline, 3-months post-randomisation and 6-months post randomisation separately to examine if any characteristics appear to be associated with the presence or absence of data. As the primary strategy to handle missing data, the unadjusted analysis of continuous study variables will use a likelihood-based approach as the primary approach to deal with missing data. This approach assumes that the probability of missing data on the study variable is not related to the missing data but to some of the observed measured data in the model. That is, it assumes that the data are Missing at Random."

Fig. 9.1 Excerpt from HOMESIDE Statistical Analysis Plan

appropriately combining results obtained from each of them (Jakobsen et al., 2017; Nooraee et al., 2018).

Finally, the *likelihood-based* approach may be used to replace missing items with a value. It is based on the theory about estimating models (recovering parameters from data samples) rather than specifying (constructing) models (Frey, 2018). Through specific multilevel and structural equation models, estimates are calculated of what values are "most likely". To illustrate how planned treatment of missing data is detailed in a SAP, I have taken an extract out of our HOMESIDE SAP (Fig. 9.1).

References

Baker, F. A., Bloska, J., Stensæth, K., Wosch, T., Bukowska, A., Braat, S., Sousa, T., Tamplin, J., Clark, I. N., Lee, Y.-E. C., Clarke, P., Lautenschlager, N., & Odell-Miller, H. (2019). HOMESIDE: A home-based family caregiver-delivered music intervention for people living with dementia: Protocol of a randomised controlled trial. *British Medical Journal Open*. https://doi.org/10.1136/bmjopen-2019-031332

Baker, F. A., Lee, Y.-E. C., Sousa, T. V., Stretton-Smith, P. A., Tamplin, J., Sveinsdottir, V., Geretsegger, M., Wake, J. D., Assmus, J., Christian Gold, C. (2022). Clinical effectiveness of Music Interventions for Dementia and Depression in Elderly care (MIDDEL) in the Australian cohort: Pragmatic cluster-randomised controlled trial. *The Lancet Healthy Longevity*, *3*(3), e153–e165.

DeMets, D. L., Cook, T. D., & Buhr, K. A. (2017). Guidelines for statistical analysis plans. *Journal of the American Medical Association*, *318*(23), 2301–2303. https://doi.org/10.1001/jama.2017.18954

Finfer, S., & Bellomo, R. (2009). Why publish statistical analysis plans?—Editorial. *Critical Care and Resuscitation*, *11*(1), 5–6. https://doi.org/10.3316/informit.514015812932860

Frey, B. (2018). *The SAGE encyclopedia of educational research, measurement, and evaluation* (Vols. 1–4). SAGE Publications. https://doi.org/10.4135/9781506326139

Gamble, C., Krishan, A., Stocken, D., Lewis, S., Juszczak, E., Doré, C., Williamson, P. R., Altman, D. G., Montgomery, A., Lim, P., Berlin, J., Senn, S., Day, S., Barbachano, Y., & Loder, E. (2017). Guidelines for the content of Statistical Analysis Plans in clinical trials. *Journal of the American Medical Association*, *318*(23), 2337–2343. https://doi.org/10.1001/jama.2017.18556

Golubovic, J., Neerland, B. E., Simpso, M.R., & Baker, F. A. (Under Review). Live and recorded music interventions for management of delirium symptoms in acute geriatric patients: Theoretical framework and protocol for a randomised feasibility trial. *BMC Geriatrics*.

Hiemstra, B., Keus, F., Wetterslev, J., Gluud, C., & van der Horst, I. C. C. (2019). DEBATE-statistical analysis plans for observational studies. *BMC Medical Research Methodology*, *19*(1), 1–10. https://doi.org/10.1186/s12874-019-0879-5

Jakobsen, J. C., Gluud, C., & Wetterslev, J. (2017). When and how should multiple imputation be used for handling missing data in randomised clinical trials—A practical guide with flowcharts. *BMC Medical Research Methodology*, *17*, 162. https://doi.org/10.1186/s12874-017-0442-1

Jorgensen, A. W., Lundstrom, L. H., Wetterslev, J., Astrup, A., & Gotzsche, P. C. (2014). Comparison of results from different imputation techniques for missing data from an anti-obesity drug trial. *PLoS ONE*, *9*(11), e111964.

Kang, H. (2013). The prevention and handling of the missing data. *Korean Journal of Anesthesiology*, *64*(5), 402–406. https://doi.org/10.4097/kjae.2013.64.5.402

Kumar, A., & Chakraborty, B. S. (2016). Interim analysis: A rational approach of decision making in clinical trial. *Journal of Advanced Pharmaceutical Technology & Research, 7*(4), 118–122. https://doi.org/10.4103/2231-4040.191414

Lesaffre, E. (2008). Superiority, equivalence, and non-inferiority trials. *Bulletin of the Hospital for Joint Diseases, 66*(2), 150–154.

Mack, C., Su, Z., & Westreich, D. (2018). *Managing missing data in patient registries: Addendum to registries for evaluating patient outcomes: A user's guide* (3rd ed.) (Internet). Agency for Healthcare Research and Quality (US); Types of Missing Data. https://www.ncbi.nlm.nih.gov/books/NBK493614/. Accessed 30 July 2022.

Nooraee, N., Molenberghs, G., Ormel, J., & Van den Heuvel, E. R. (2018). Strategies for handling missing data in longitudinal studies with questionnaires. *Journal of Statistical Computation and Simulation, 88*(17), 3415–3436. https://doi.org/10.1080/00949655.2018.1520854

The Lancet. (2010). Should protocols for observational research be registered? *Lancet, 375*(9712), 1.

Thomas, L., & Peterson, E. D. (2012). The value of Statistical Analysis Plans in observational research: Defining high-Quality research from the start. *Journal of the American Medical Association, 308*(8), 773–774. https://doi.org/10.1001/jama.2012.9502

Yuan, I., Topjian, A. A., Kurth, C. D., Kirschen, M. P., Ward, C. G., Zhang, B., & Mensinger, J. L. (2019). Guide to the statistical analysis plan. *Pediatric Anesthesia, 29*(3), 237. https://doi.org/doi.org/10.1111/pan.13576

CHAPTER 10

Development of a Knowledge Translation and Exchange Plan

OUR ETHICAL RESPONSIBILITY TO DISSEMINATE

The 2013 version of the Declaration of Helsinki states that "Researchers, authors, sponsors, editors and publishers all have ethical obligations with regard to the publication and dissemination of the results of research. Researchers have a duty to make publicly available the results of their research on human participants and are accountable for the completeness and accuracy of their reports" (World Medical Association, 2013). Importantly, the WHO statement on Public Disclosure of Clinical Trial Results states, "at a minimum, main findings of clinical trials, positive or negative, are to be submitted for publication in a peer reviewed journal within 12 months of study completion and are to be published through an open access mechanism unless there is a specific reason why open access cannot be used, or otherwise made available publicly at most within 24 months of study completion" (WHO, 2005). And lastly, in a recent study about participants' perceptions and preferences for research dissemination, participants expressed that researchers should disseminate the findings because it implicitly honours the contract made between the researcher and participants and validates that their participation has made a contribution to knowledge and that it "mattered" (Purvis et al., 2017).

All researchers want to get their work published and share their findings, however, many researchers do not consider the dissemination avenues and timeline until late in the project, often while they are undergoing the statistical analysis of the data. Certainly, that was how I operated when I was a novice researcher, until I began to appreciate the need for a well-designed knowledge translation and exchange plan. And, the dissemination strategy needs to go beyond the traditional approaches such as publications in academic journals as these have limited reach and utility for those who need it—patients, families, and the community (Long et al., 2017). One recent study found that only 27% of researchers disseminated the results of their clinical trials to those who participated in it (Schroter et al., 2019).

Consideration of a dissemination plan is the responsibility of the entire research team, not just the principal investigator. Large clinical trials may have established a publications steering committee whose membership comprises of some or all of the lead investigators. Their responsibility is to establish and then implement written guidelines for vetting papers emanating from the trial. This procedure for planning, reviewing, and approving all scientific publications (papers and abstracts) prior to submission is to ensure they are accurate (i.e. align with protocol), not duplicative, and respect International Committee of Medical Journal Editors (ICMJE) authorship guidelines.

What Is and Why Implement Knowledge Translation and Exchange?

Before I begin to outline some approaches to developing the Knowledge Translation and Exchange (KTE) plan, an overview of what knowledge translation and exchange means in the context of health research is needed. This "buzz phrase" is a term that now permeates the health research methodology literature and there is an expectation that KTE is implemented throughout the study, not just at the project's end. Indeed, most major grant schemes these days include KTE as one of its assessable selection criteria.

The Canadian Institutes of Health Research (2009) defines KTE as "the dynamic and iterative process that includes the synthesis, dissemination, exchange, and ethically sound application of knowledge, to improve health, provide more effective health services and products, and strengthen the healthcare system". This implies that knowledge gained from research outcomes is translated and communicated to a range of stakeholders with the hope of uptake in real world practice. In the context of the creative arts therapies, the KTE is a process whereby we share our knowledge with decision-makers and communities to either influence policy, help health professionals recognise the contribution we can make to quality health care, and to facilitate improved understanding by the consumers so that they may be more likely to self-refer.

The KTE is a reciprocal process—not a one-way process from researcher imparting knowledge to stakeholders—hence the term "exchange" whereby the research team engage with decision-makers, communities, and practitioners, to ensure that the benefits of the intervention for end-users (our creative arts therapies clients) are considered. At the same time, the needs of policy-makers with political pressures need to be balanced alongside the research evidence (Armstrong et al., 2008). Almost invariably, every creative arts therapist who engages in clinical trials, is not doing so just to generate money, but hopes their outcomes will result in funding or policy changes. In essence, this motivation underpins (and therefore biases) our design and the targeted outcomes but we need to be aware that when using the research evidence to influence policy, this needs to be considered in the context of the bigger political picture.

Dissemination Development Plan

When developing the dissemination plan, it is helpful to consider these six key components—(1) research findings and products, (2) end-users, (3) dissemination partners, (4) communication approaches, (5) evaluation of dissemination, and the (6) the dissemination work plan.

Research Findings and Products

The more complex the clinical trial, the more findings and/or products the research team may have generated that need dissemination and the more diverse audiences that may be benefit from the dissemination process. The first task therefore is to define exactly what findings and outputs are key to share. Here, it is important to highlight that outputs can extend beyond just the research findings but can be broader contributions to the research community, healthcare community, policy-makers, and consumers. Here are some examples that the research team may consider:

1. *Developed research measuring tools or methodologies.* As we evolve as a dynamic collective group of creative arts therapy researchers, in

addition to developing and testing the effectiveness of our interventions, we may be concurrently developing different methodologies that are both findful and robust means to measure the therapeutic effects. I offer three examples, although there are undoubtedly many more. In our MIDDEL trial (Baker et al., 2022) where we tested two different music interventions on the depression and psychiatric symptoms of people living with dementia, we developed a set of carefully designed intervention fidelity checklists (Baker, Tamplin, et al., 2019). These checklists were created to to ensure that the interventions in the MIDDEL trial were delivered as intended and that the two interventions were sufficiently differentiated so as to capture the true effects of each (see Chapter 8). Not only did this increase the transparency and integrity of our study, but by publishing the strategies and processes we engaged in to develop them, other researchers could draw on these when developing their own set of fidelity checklists.

The second example was a publication that emerged from within the Remini-Sing trial (Tamplin et al., 2018). This mixed methods study involved interviewing people living with dementia who had participated in a dementia choir program. We believe that the voices of people living with dementia were mostly absent from music therapy studies, so we developed a methodology and subsequent guidelines for implementing accessible and inclusive interviews (Thompson et al., 2021). Again, publishing these guidelines is something that future researchers can utilise to inform their own study methodology.

The last example was the development and validation of a validated assessment tool that measures how "meaningful" an experience of songwriting is for the people who engage in songwriting as part of their therapy process. We hypothesised that those who derived greater meaning from participation, were more likely to have larger therapeutic outcomes when compared with those who found the songwriting process less personally meaningful. As there was no existing measure, we needed to develop and validate a measure (Baker et al., 2015). This tool has been since used by other researchers in research and in clinical practice.

2. *Intervention protocols.* While study protocols are a standard part of the dissemination plan, less common are published protocols of the interventions. Study protocol papers rarely have the space needed to

go in depth into the theory underpinning the intervention and the detailed approach so that it could be replicated in clinical practice. One example of such a publication was the songwriting and identity intervention protocol developed for people post brain injury. The publication outlined the concepts of past, present, and future identities that people who had sustained a brain injury needed to integrate into their sense of self-identity. Our publication explained how we integrated these concepts into our intervention protocol to test how exploring past, present, and future identities through narrative songwriting, could impact on post-intervention identity (Tamplin et al., 2016). This publication was directed at clinicians who may want to incorporate this intervention protocol in their clinical work.

3. *Cost-benefit, cost-effectiveness, and health economics of trials.* Several trials in the creative arts therapies are beginning to embed health economics components to their trials. These outcomes are important to publish because they may make powerful arguments that can influence funders of creative arts services in the future. Some examples include Chlan et al. (2018) and Park et al. (2016), and other trials currently underway (Baker, Bloska, et al., 2019; Gold et al., 2019). It's important to note that to undertake a comprehensive cost-effectiveness analysis, a qualified health economics researcher should be recruited to the research team (see Chapter 4).

4. *Perspectives of consumers, families, and staff.* Like cost-effectiveness papers, it is increasingly common for researchers to disseminate the perspectives of consumers, families, and staff about (a) participating in research and (b) how they experienced participation in the intervention itself. Dissemination of the key measures can occur in academic publications (e.g. Lee, Stretton-Smith, et al., 2022), at conferences targeting consumers and their families, or in the media—radio, television, online print media (e.g. The Conversation [https://theconversation.com/songwriting-as-solace-i-live-in-the-same-body-but-it-cant-talk-to-me-any-more-59154?utm_medium=email&utm_campaign=Latest%20from%20The%20Conversation%20for%20May%2012%202016%20-%204839&utm_content=Latest%20from%20The%20Conversation%20for%20May%2012%202016%20-%204839+CID_38173413147cc5d674696144215ef9fa&utm_source=campaign_monitor&utm_term=Songwriting%20as%20solace%20I%20live%20in%20the%20same%20body%20but%20it%20cant%20talk%20to%20me%20any%20more]), or social media.

5. *Profile or demographic data.* While outcomes of an intervention are useful, sometimes more detailed demographic data (baseline data) can be helpful beyond intervention research for understanding the general health profile of a population. In our MIDDEL study, because we had recruited more than 300 residents with dementia from 24 different care home units across Melbourne, we were able to report on baselines data that highlighted the profile of these residents. Data such as mean age, gender balance, ethnicity, severity of dementia, and other relevant data were made available so that others interested in studying this population, could draw on our baseline data to inform them of what the profile of this population is in residential aged care in Australia (Lee, Sousa, et al., 2022).

6. *Management of clinical trials.* With the increasing complexity of clinical trials, any published data that can assist researchers in planning and implementing a study is helpful. There are whole journals that focus on communicating trial methodology. Given the effort researchers invest in implementing a trial, it can be rewarding (but more importantly useful), to publish the strategies, challenges, and outcomes associated with implementing methodologies to manage a trial. I offer two examples. The first involves the reporting of resource use in recruiting and assessing participants. The MIDDEL study systematically collected data on the number of phone calls, time spent assessing participants, time spent discussing participants with staff, and the time spent following up on retrieving consent forms, etc. (Baker et al., 2020). Our main finding was that two-thirds of the time spent on site in residential aged care was in "waiting" for staff to be free to communicate with us. Similarly, it took an average of 45 days to receive informed consent from next of kin from the first contact until receiving the signed form. This type of information is helpful for those planning to implement a trial in residential aged care.

Identify End-Users

Before we can consider *how* to communicate to different audiences, we need to consider *who* we want to communicate with and develop the dissemination plan accordingly. When doing so, it can be helpful to engage the community of stakeholders to ensure sufficient reach and that all audiences are considered (Cunningham-Erves et al., 2020). Including consumers (patients/families) in the development of the plan will assist in translating the findings into language that is clear and understandable to a lay audience. This will increase the changes of better adoption and circulation of the research findings (McNichol & Grimshaw, 2014).

In preparing the list of end-users, consider those beyond the patients and clients that will benefit. These can range from the clinicians who will implement the interventions with the target clinical population, the organisations who are considering employing a creative arts therapist, governments, or health insurance companies considering funding the therapy, and academics who want to build on the research.

When preparing this list, try to be as specific as possible because how, where and when you disseminate will be dependent upon who you want to share knowledge with. For example, do you want your findings to share with general practitioners or more specialist physicians such as gerontologists or oncologists. These audiences will be likely reached through different avenues. And when preparing the list, consider what your audiences would want to know. Again, consider the difference between what a nurse, patient, and funder will want to know.

Another consideration is what recent or future events might help or hinder the interest of your audiences. For example, a change in government or health policy may present an opportunity to disseminate or suggest a different approach or avenue for dissemination. If you have a public and patient involvement committee participating in your research project (see Chapter 3), involving them in your dissemination plan can make your plan more targeted and likely to succeed in knowledge translation. And finally, consider what enablers and barriers your end-users may encounter when wanting to access your findings. How will the audience know to "trust" you and what findings you present?

COLLABORATING WITH PARTNERS FOR DISSEMINATION

Maximising the reach of your findings—locally, nationally, and globally—will need support from different types of partners. These partners can be formal partners—academics, industry partners, professional organisations—or can be informal networks. Every health profession including the creative arts therapies have what is known as "opinion leaders", people who are good at, and committed to, disseminating important findings. Organisational partners can take the form of advocacy groups, healthcare providers, and professional bodies. Draw on whatever networks you have to hand, and ask for assistance from those in your network to link you in with others that may have an interest in supporting the dissemination of your research findings.

When approaching them for support, consider how your research findings can advance their organisation's vision, mission, and operation. In other words, "what's in it for them?" If you can frame your research in a way that shows how the findings positively impact their organisation, this may be a way to garner their support in the dissemination process. I offer one example of art therapists working with children who have attention deficit disorder. If an art therapy after school program has been shown to improve focused attention and regulate behaviour, discussing the possibility of advocacy groups disseminating this via their members may lead to parents putting pressure on schools to employ an art therapist. When such results do happen, the advocacy group can highlight how they supported the dissemination of best practice to families affected by attention deficit disorder.

Communicating Your Message

Communicating and interacting with different types of audiences is challenging. As academics/researchers, we are used to communicating our findings to the research community. But we have little training in expanding our communication style and approach to different audiences—discipline specific and interdisciplinary academics, politicians, healthcare managers, public and private health insurance management, general practitioners, the media, our client groups, and our creative arts therapy practitioners. Communicating with each group has a different purpose, demands a different narrative, and a different use of language.

Increasingly, universities are providing training in research translation and impact and I would encourage all researchers wanting to have community impact, to enrol in a workshop or training session if one is offered. Finding champions of your research from the different audiences is also helpful. When preparing your messaging, consult with them on your approach and hone the message until it targets' their needs and level of understanding. Involving consumers and stakeholders in the development of the messaging will help ensure they are culturally appropriate, have readability/comprehensibility, are engaging, jargon-free, and are effective in conveying the content (Armstrong et al., 2008; Kulig & Westlund, 2015; Purvis et al., 2017).

Evaluation of Your Dissemination Plan

Consider your dissemination strategy as a long-term activity. It's not something you do as a "one off" activity, but messaging needs to be repeated to maximise the opportunity for it to translate into change. Similarly, the more often you present your findings and in more varied ways, the better you get at communicating these and pitching them to the right audience. For example, I was presenting a 5-minute "pitch" to potential investors to attract some seed funding to develop our minimal viable product—our MATCH app. Investors were interested in how MATCH would solve a problem, what the size of the problem was, who would use it, how it was different to other solutions, who would buy it, what was our model for reaching those who would need it, etc. This was a completely different way of presenting the research than what I had been used to. It took a series of practice-runs over three months to hone my messaging, taking on feedback from every person who I presented it to. In the end, it was sharp, snappy, and business like—a totally different feel to anything I have presented before.

An important component of the dissemination plan is to decide on a method of evaluating the success of your dissemination efforts. You might collect data such as the number of website hits, the number of people attending a webinar, the circulation of a trade magazine. That said, the number "reached" is not necessarily an indicator of the number who took something meaningful away from the knowledge exchange activity however numbers of those accessing the information goes someway to evaluate reach.

Perhaps the greatest sign that a dissemination plan is working well is to see a change in the sector. This could be a greater uptake of the intervention within an already existing creative arts therapy service or greater demand for services from organisations or clients not currently receiving it. More significant would be a change in government policy or funding models. It is unlikely that a single creative arts therapy study could have such transformative influence on policy changes, but certainly collective evidence generated from multiple trials is more likely to lead to systemic change.

Strategies and Considerations for Implementing KTE

To increase the reach of your findings, utilise a broad range of channels. Aside from the typical journal publication, consider communicating findings on websites, at meetings and conferences, trade magazines, through organisational bulletins, special interest groups, public seminars, white papers, media, interest group listservs, and social media including twitter, podcasts, and YouTube clips. However, when considering a spectrum of channels, it is important to consider which audience uses which channels and tailor the communication style to that audience. Further, do not use all the channels because they "exist", be selective about which ones are most likely to reach those you want to reach. I now outline a few strategies to consider as you draft your plan.

1. *Policy changing strategies.* First and foremost, when considering policy-changing objectives, the research team can engage decision-makers and policy-makers in a series of face-to-face meetings to discuss the findings, the relevance of these for the sector or healthcare context, and provide opportunities for a dialogue and development of a plan for systemic change (Marin-Gonzalezm et al., 2017). There may be an element of educating these policy-makers about what our creative arts therapies do, before the implications and implementation potential of the research evidence can be understood. It is important to think of building change incrementally, suggestions for radical change are unlikely to be received well. It can be helpful to set up the dialogue to highlight how implementing your research findings in practice addresses one of their key needs or problems.

    Case example. Disseminating MIDDEL findings to Health Department policy-makers. I began a dialogue with policy leaders of the public sector funded residential aged care homes following the published findings from the MIDDEL paper. I first approached the minister for ageing and invited him to have a meeting with me to discuss the crisis the aged care sector was facing and how introducing music therapy to residential aged care homes in Victoria could contribute to solving the problems they were encountering. In my brief email introduction, I used a specific strategy to pique his interest.

(1) State facts about the core problems facing the sector.
(2) Outline what the sector would look like if those problems were lessened or eliminated.
(3) Introduce the concept of music therapy and highlight the findings from the research I conducted and how it directly addresses the problem (including stating which health outcomes it specifically addressed).
(4) Outline the cost savings of introducing music therapy.[1]
(5) Detail the costs of investing in music therapy, highlighting the cost-benefit.
(6) Highlight the added value of introducing an evidence-based intervention.
(7) Include some consumer quotes where possible.
(8) Sum up with a statement about the opportunity presented to them.

In addition to the face-to-face meetings, reaching stakeholders through short reports, booklets, leaflets, and infographics that are short, succinct, and easily digestible, can increase the likelihood of your message being received and remembered (Marın-Gonzalezm et al., 2017).

2. *Capacity building.* Part of our responsibility as creative arts therapy researchers is to build the expertise and capacity of the clinicians who are having face-to-face contact with clients. There is a missed opportunity if we fail to improve the knowledge, skills, and expertise of our creative arts therapies community by translating findings into practice guidelines and subsequently disseminating them to clinicians. The guidelines might include descriptions of the characteristics of clients that are best suited to the intervention, detailed intervention descriptions, and recommendations for implementation. But this capacity building potential can extend beyond our own disciplines (Armstrong et al., 2008). We can engage with the broader healthcare team and family carers to "educate" them on what our creative arts therapies interventions can achieve. We may even provide guidance on how they can utilise the findings

---

[1] This was addressed by the notion that a reduction in scores on the NPI-Q agitation item by just one point, would reduce care costs by 8%. Our data showed a decrease in this item by a mean of 1.2.

to improve the provision of their own health care. Again, using our MIDDEL study as an example, we actively sought audiences where we could educate music therapy clinicians about the finding that "singing" as a music activity, seems to have more impact on depression than other music activities such as improvisation and movement to music. We promoted this finding through our closed Facebook special interest groups, at music therapy conferences, and through bulletin announcements disseminated by The Australian Music Therapy Association. We also presented these findings at dementia and ageing conferences. Here, our messaging was different to tailored towards our clinicians. We wanted to highlight the finding that those participants with more severe dementia responded to a greater degree than those with less severe dementia. Therefore, our messaging was focused on referrals emphasising that when resources (music therapist's hours) are limited, referrals to music therapy should be directed towards those residents with dementia who are more progressed in their disease.

3. *Web-based and electronic print media.* In an era when information is mostly going to be discovered via the World Wide Web, it is important for researchers to disseminate their findings through electronic mediums. One way to disseminate is through the use of a project website. Not only can it be helpful during the project to give the public an update on project milestones, but it can also be an excellent medium for disseminating the key findings of a project. Given websites are publicly available, it is critical to focus on devising messages that can be understood by a layperson. Branding including the creation of a meaningful and engaging logo and acronym, can make locating the research findings easier for the public (Kulig & Westlund, 2015).

4. *Creative mediums.* Aside from web-based and electronic print media, there are several other potential mediums where researchers can report their findings. The rise of social media as a novel tool to disseminate is increasing. Social media—Facebook, LinkedIn, twitter, podcasts, and videos (YouTube and Vimeo)—can raise public awareness of research, enable interaction between researchers and the lay public, and can stimulate discussion and debate between members of the public (Deeken et al., 2020). It has been suggested that social media can result in increased readership of articles and

therefore increased citations in a variety of fields (e.g. Eysenbach, 2011).

When considering providing summaries of findings to the study participants, Purvis et al. (2017) found that the mode of sharing findings differed dependent upon the age of participants. In general, younger participants preferred email or social media as the best medium for sharing findings while older participants preferred mail or face-to-face communication. While no recent studies on this issue have been undertaken, as a consequence of the COVID-19 pandemic, in my experience in working with older people, this preference for mail versus email and social media, is fast changing. Importantly, participants have indicated that dissemination should be provided in multiple forms to accommodate differences in preference.

For those client groups where there is limited cognitive capacity to read and understand textual content, creating short films or video clips with the key messages in simple language, can make the findings accessible. The messages will be even more understandable if there is the capacity to include participant voice within the clips. A note of caution, however. From an ethical perspective, it is important to consider that consent to share participants' experiences does not assume a "for all time" consent. So, using participant voice should be time-limited and discussed with the participant at the time of gaining permission to use their quote.

Authorship and Publishing

For many researchers at any stage of their career, publishing together with collaborators can be a rewarding and stimulating experience. However, it can be fraught with challenges, stress, and conflict if not dealt with in a collegial way. I have processed my own feelings around having been excluded from a manuscript where I felt I had contributed to the design and interpretation of the findings. Similarly, I needed to process my response to a scenario where I felt my contribution was not recognised enough as evidenced by where I was placed in the authorship order. While never having spoken up about this with the research lead, when I reflect now, having a good publication dialogue ahead of the drafting of the manuscript can avoid such scenarios and potential conflict further down the track.

Who is eligible to be an author has attracted a lot of debate and it can be confusing for the novice creative arts therapies researcher to navigate this, especially when engaging in interdisciplinary research with seasoned researchers. In general, anyone who has made a substantial contribution to a research project throughout its implementation (Katib, 2020) should be invited to become an author. The International Committee for Medical Journal Editors (2019) proposed that the criteria for authorship be that authors make (1) Substantial contributions to the conception and design of the work; or the acquisition, analysis, or interpretation of data for the work; AND (2) Drafting the work or revising it critically for important intellectual content; AND (3) Final approval of the version to be published; AND (4) Agreement to be accountable for all aspects of the work in ensuring that questions related to the accuracy or integrity of any part of the work are appropriately investigated and resolved. While these criteria are still used today, there has been some critique on whether all four criteria need to be satisfied to qualify for authorship. Sethy (2020) offered an alternative and a more transparent way to identify how to determine what the relative contributions are for an author by scoring authors across a 5-point system.

- Concept development (4)—initiating the new ideas for the research and assessing its "validity, genuineness, and appropriateness" to generate a research question that is important to answer.
- Research Design (4)—makes decisions on the methodology and outcome measures that answer the objectives and are feasible (timeframes, resources, practical issues).
- Research supervision (2)—supervising the whole team and supporting junior researchers.
- Study material collection (paid job) (1)—collecting data as instructed by researchers and study protocol.
- Data collection (paid job) (1)—preparing data collection materials and/or collecting data as instructed by researchers and study protocol.
- Data collection by the researcher (3)—designing data collection materials and collecting data.
- Data management (3)—designing the database so that data is labelled and categorised appropriately. It requires knowledge about the research questions and design.

- Data Analysis and interpretation (4)—makes decisions about analysis approaches and later how to interpret whether the results support the hypotheses.
- Literature review (5)—prepares the review to justify the research questions and methodology and to contextualise it within the broader field.
- Writing the paper (5)—bringing together the components of the research to write a report according to reporting guidelines (e.g. SPIRIT).
- Revising the article (4)—contributes to revising the article based on reviewer feedback.
- English language editing services (copy editing and proofreading)—(paid job) (1).

When assigning these scores, those scoring 1, should be acknowledged in the acknowledgements section. Those scoring 2 (minimal contribution), 3 (significant contribution), 4 (major contribution), and 5 (core contribution) should all be included as authors. Calculating the total scores can be a tool to decide author order when using Katib's (2020) approach of "relative contribution".

Sethy's (2020) system is helpful when trying to decide the order of authorship. While in theory, all authors should be credited equally to the project which is the result of a whole team effort, this is not the case. Indeed, the first author is the most coveted position because of its increased visibility (Katib, 2020). This author is often the project leader and because of the emotional investment in the project, is the person to drive, lead, and take responsibility for the manuscript (Duncan, 1999). This leadership involves coordinating the drafting of the manuscript including holding meetings, keeping records of all dated copies of drafts. The first author also typically edits the work so there is a consistent writing style and seeing endorsement of all authors about the final manuscript prior to submission. The first author is often responsible for also checking the copyedited proof ensuring that there are no errors or that any editorial changes made by the publisher do not change the content or meaning (Duncan, 1999). This includes checking tables and included data. The last author is often taken by the project leader (chief investigator). While not always the case, this person is often the person who either conceptualises the project and/or designs substantial (if not all) aspects of the study design.

While the first and last author position is relatively easy to determine, how does one decide the remaining order. Katib (2020) pose three models. The first, and perhaps most common is the relative contribution where the author who has contributed the most substantially to the research and drafting of the article becomes the first author, with all others listed in descending order of contribution. This is where Sethy's (2020) system can be helpful. This is definitely the approach I have used most consistently throughout my career. The second approach is the alphabetical list where authors are listed alphabetically. This approach is often used for projects involving large numbers of researchers. I have also used this approach (see Baker, Bloska, et al., 2019). The third approach is the negotiated order, where aside from the first and last author, there is no general agreement, and the team leads a discussion to make those decisions.

As Sethy (2020) outline, determining the relative contribution to the project as a whole is helpful in deciding who warrants authorship on a paper. That said, each author does have a responsibility in contributing to the manuscript. Duncan (1999) argues that contributing to the drafting or revising of the manuscript is the responsibility of authors, and that "just showing up for meetings but not contributing intellectually" is not good enough. Duncan likens this to "being a potential co-owner of that fictitious house and not knowing how many rooms it contained". She recommends that the first author ensure that every author dates and initials a final copy prior to submission to highlight the need for accountability and that there is proof the final manuscript has had final approval by all authors.

Transparency in author contributions has been made easier with the increasing use of a contributor statement published at the end of the manuscript. In these statements, there is a clear outline of who did what as part of the project and write up of the manuscript. An example of this has been taken from our recent publication in (Baker et al., 2022). It can be seen clearly from the statement who did what in this project.

> *Contributors:* CG^2 took the initiative for the study; FAB, YCL, MG, and JA contributed to development of concept design; FAB obtained funding and led the implementation of the trial; FAB, JT, and YCL developed fidelity measures, intervention manuals, and trained interventionists; YCL supervised assessors; JT and FAB supervised interventionists; YCL and PSS

> liaised with industry partners; FAB, YCL, and PSS were involved in setting up the study conduct in each site. FB, JT, YCL and PSS completed fidelity checks; CG, MG, JDW, JA and VS were responsible for data management activities; CG and JA conducted the main statistical analysis; TVS and PC completed the health economics analysis; FAB, CG, YCL, PSS, and TVS drafted the manuscript; JT, VS, MG, JDW, and JA helped drafting the manuscript. All authors approved the final version of the manuscript.

Like all aspects of research implementation, decisions about the order of authorship should be decided early, preferably no later than the beginning of the first draft of the article (Duncan, 1999). It can be helpful to have a meeting to discuss author order, make decisions about the roles of each author, and if needed, write a contract. Identifying the team member who has had the least to do with the project, can take a more objective stance and is a great person to review the whole first draft, identifying what makes sense, what is missing, where further elaborations are needed and where there is too much detail. Being able to link the discussion points and interpretations back to the analysed data is also an important role for someone who is a bit more distant.

The more authors there are, the more difficult these discussions are. Further, the team should be open to additional discussions as the project progresses about the order of authorship if the researchers' roles and contributions shift over time. Again, this process can be quite a delicate one and requires the principal investigator address this with a degree of reflexivity and sensitivity. Reflecting on my own experiences of feeling overlooked helps in being responsive and anticipating uneasy feelings among group members. Nevertheless, these difficult conversations are inevitable and necessary at some point with a goal of avoiding crises later in the process.

When leading a large project that may have multiple research workstreams, different investigators are leading and overseeing different components, and there are likely to be multiple publication outputs. If this is the case, at the commencement of the project, the team can begin to decide on the types of outputs and identify specific journals that might be appropriate to publish in. From here, an egalitarian strategy can be to discuss who would be best to lead the particular publications ensuring

---

[2] Initials of authors.

that all members of the team have an opportunity to lead manuscripts if they wish to. This part of the dissemination plan can be a living document and should be reviewed and when necessary, revised regularly at team meetings.

Developing an overall project publication policy and/or investigator contract can be helpful, making sure that all investigators have an opportunity to have input into the policy/contract and that the final version is agreed on and approved by all investigators. Duncan (1999) suggests that a contract should outline the expectations of investigators wanting to participate in a manuscript as well as what consequences there are for not meeting those. The contracts may include which team members will be responsible for different aspects of the work, how people will work together, planning deadlines around drafts, any agreement around rotation of authorship, plans for mediation if needed, and the ways the principal investigator manages non-compliance with the workload (e.g. should this person be recognised as an author, a contributor or be asked to step down entirely from the project).

A policy I developed for the MATCH project before the first participant enrolment was as follows:

> **Case example. Publication Policy for Music Attuned Technology for Care via eHealth Publication**
> This policy and procedure document was developed and agreed upon by the 10 MATCH chief investigators.
> **Procedure**
> The policy is designed to have a clear process for deciding authorship and for handling non-compliance.
>
> 1. All 10 chief investigators who have had substantial input into the initial conceptual development and methodological decisions at the time of developing the proposal will have the option to opt in or opt out of manuscripts arising from this work irrespective of workstream. If they choose to opt in, they must attend meetings chaired by first author and agree to contribute to the manuscript as agreed upon with the first author.
> 2. The first author of the manuscript is responsible for:

(a) Notifying all chief investigators of the intent of the manuscript, the proposed journal for submission, and the expected timeframe/deadlines to complete first draft and second draft. The first author will also request receipt of the notification and a deadline for chief investigators to make a preliminary decision to opt in or opt out.
(b) Deciding and inviting relevant associate investigators and other doctoral students or research fellows involved in the project to join as co-authors. The first author must notify them of the proposed journal submission, and the expected timeframe/deadlines to complete first draft and second draft. The first author will also request receipt of the notification and a deadline for associate investigators and other invited researchers to make a preliminary decision to opt in or opt out.
(c) Organise an initial meeting with the proposed authors and subsequent meetings.
(d) Facilitate a discussion on roles and responsibilities of the drafting of the manuscript and authorship order.
(e) Coordinate the drafting of the manuscript including sending reminders to authors on upcoming agreed deadlines.
(f) Coordinate proofing and checking references of submission.
(g) Coordinate the sign off by all authors prior to submission.
(h) Draft letter to the editor and submit manuscript for review.
(i) Coordinate any revisions required.
(j) Proof the manuscript and return with any corrections.
(k) Sign off on corrected proof.
(l) Coordinate copyright with publishers and organise payment of fees for open access publications.

3. Discussions about order of authorship should be led by the first author. The first author should

   (a) Hold an initial meeting to discuss roles and responsibilities of each confirmed author.
   (b) Collaboratively evaluate the contribution of each author using an *Authorship Contribution Checklist*.
   (c) Formalise agreement on authorship order either through meeting minutes or by email.

Disputes over authorship should be mediated by a suitable person not directly involved in the study. This could be a person nominated by

> the Chair of the Advisory Committee or the Faculty Associate Dean (Research) or equivalent. Where resolution cannot be reached, the matter will be referred to the University's central Office for Research Ethics and Integrity.

Publication Bias

Publication integrity is an aspect of dissemination that needs to be considered and one that has been discussed at length in the health research literature. We know that not all research makes it to publication. Similarly, some authors have been known to withhold some data from publication and only present the findings that are positive (bias). What is and is not published, can be influenced from several spheres—researchers/authors, journal editors, reviewers, funding bodies, and universities (Bassler et al., 2016) which are worthy of a brief mention here so that researchers can keep these factors in mind while developing their research dissemination plan.

The first factor which may influence publication bias is the concept of publish or perish, a phenomenon that has permeated the sector (but thankfully) there is a shift to recognition of quality over quantity. Researchers may experience a range of pressures to publish a lot of manuscripts and to publish fast. This pressure may be internally or externally driven. Internally, the researchers may want to increase their visibility, reputation, and standing in the field which has flow-on effects to securing tenured creative arts therapies university positions or to increased access to funding opportunities (Katib, 2020). In many research funding schemes such as research fellowships, up to 40% of the assessment criteria is based on the assessment of previous track-record of applicants. In other words, without a strong publication record, your chances of securing a grant are low. Externally, driven factors can relate to university pressures such as a minimum number of peer reviewed publications per year (often averaged over a 3–5-year period) or the expectations from funding bodies that publications will be an expected output from previously funded research (Bassler et al., 2016).

Another factor impacting publication integrity is the notion that novel research findings are desirable and more likely to be rewarded by being accepted for publication. Editors want to publish good research, but they also want to publish research that is innovative, likely to be highly cited (as this reinforces the journal's standing), and increasingly will attract media interest. Consequently, authors may look to publish only the research that is considered sufficiently interesting to editors (Bassler et al., 2016; Katib, 2020) while neglecting to report "all" the findings, hence bias. Related to this, is the increase in open access publishing and that journal's stand to make money from publications. In 2021, several journals had fees as high as US$4,000+ to publish in their journals. There is therefore a financial interest in publishing research, and may lead to a reduction in research quality.

Conclusion

Knowledge translation and exchange can be challenging on several levels including identifying who the main stakeholders are and what component of the research findings they may be interested in receiving. Careful planning of who, when, how, and where to disseminate will ensure maximum reach. Negotiating authorship can be a complex and sensitive issue. Authorship inclusions and discussions should be led by the lead author and be transparent, inclusive, and representative of the degree of input from each author.

References

Armstrong, R., Clark, R., Murphy, S., & Waters, E. (2008, December). Epidemiology and health policy: Strategies to support knowledge translation and exchange. *Australasian Epidemiologist, 15*(3), 24–27.

Baker, F. A., Bloska, J., Stensæth, K., Wosch, T., Bukowska, A., Braat, S., Sousa, T., Tamplin, J., Clark, I. N., Lee, Y.-E. C., Clarke, P., Lautenschlager, N., & Odell-Miller, H. (2019). HOMESIDE: A home-based family caregiver-delivered music intervention for people living with dementia: Protocol of a randomised controlled trial. *British Medical Journal Open.* https://doi.org/10.1136/bmjopen-2019-031332

Baker, F. A., Lee, Y.-E. C., Sousa, T. V., Stretton-Smith, P. A., Tamplin, J., Sveinsdottir, V., Geretsegger, M., Wake, J. D., Assmus, J., & Christian Gold, C. (2022). Clinical effectiveness of Music Interventions for Dementia and Depression in Elderly care (MIDDEL) in the Australian cohort: pragmatic cluster-randomised controlled trial. *The Lancet Healthy Longevity, 3*(3), e153–e165.

Baker, F. A., Silverman, M. J., & MacDonald, R. A. R. (2015). Reliability and validity of the Meaningfulness of Songwriting Scale (MSS) with adults on acute psychiatric and detoxification units. *Journal of Music Therapy*. https://doi.org/10.1093/jmt/thv020

Baker, F. A., Stretton-Smith, P., Sousa, T. A., Clark, I., Cotton, A., Gold, C., & Lee, Y.-E. C. (2020). Process and resource assessment in trials undertaken in residential care homes: Experiences from the Australian MIDDEL research team. *Contemporary Clinical Trials Communication*. https://doi.org/10.1016/j.conctc.2020.100675

Baker, F. A., Tamplin, J., Clark, I., Lee, Y.-E. C., Geretsegger, M., & Gold, C. (2019). Treatment fidelity in a music therapy multi-site cluster randomized control trial for people living with dementia: The MIDDEL project. *Journal of Music Therapy*. https://doi.org/10.1093/jmt/thy023

Bassler, D., Mueller, K. F., Briel, M., Kleijnen, J., Marusic, A., Wager, E., Antes, G., von Elm, E., Altman, D. G., & Meerpohl, J. J. (2016). Bias in dissemination of clinical research findings: Structured OPEN framework of what, who and why, based on literature review and expert consensus. *British Medical Journal Open, 6*(1), e010024. https://doi.org/10.1136/bmjopen-2015-010024

Canadian Institutes of Health Research. (2009). *About knowledge translation—The KT portfolio at CIHR*. Canadian Institutes of Health Research. http://www.cihr-irsc.gc.ca/e/29418.html. Accessed 8 September 2021.

Chlan, L. L., Heiderscheit, A., Skaar, D. J., & Neidecker, M. V. (2018). Economic evaluation of a patient-directed music intervention for ICU patients receiving mechanical ventilatory support. *Critical Care Medicine, 46*(9), 1430–1435.

Cunningham-Erves, J., Mayo-Gamble, T., Vaughn, Y., Hawk, J., Helms, M., Barajas, C., & Joosten, Y. (2020). Engagement of community stakeholders to develop a framework to guide research dissemination to communities. *Health Expectations, 23*, 958–968. https://doi.org/10.1111/hex.13076

Deeken, A. H., Mukhopadhyay, S., & Jiang, X. S. (2020). Social media in academics and research: 21st-century tools to turbocharge education, collaboration, and dissemination of research finding. *Histopathology, 77*, 688–699. https://doi.org/10.1111/his.14196

Duncan, A. M. (1999, May). Authorship, dissemination of research findings and related matters. *Applied Nursing Research, 12*(2), 101–106.

Eysenbach, G. (2011). Can tweets predict citations? Metrics of social impact based on Twitter and correlation with traditional metrics of scientific impact. *Journal of Medical Internet Research, 13*, e123.

Gold, C., Eickholt, J., Assmus, J., Stige, B., Wake, J. D., Baker, F. A., Tamplin, J., Clark, I. Lee, Y.-E., Jacobsen, S. J., , Ridder, H. M. O., Kreutz, G., Muthesius, D., Wosch, T., Ceccato, E., Raglio, A., Ruggeri, M., Vink, A.,

Zuidema, S., ... Geretsegger, M. (2019). Music Interventions for Dementia and Depression in ELderly care (MIDDEL): Protocol and statistical analysis plan for a multinational cluster-randomised trial. *British Medical Journal Open, 9*(3). https://doi.org/10.1136/bmjopen-2018-023436

International Committee of Medical Journal Editors (ICMJE). (2019). *Recommendations for the conduct, reporting, editing, and publication of scholarly work in medical journals.* http://www.icmje.org. Accessed 4 September 2021.

Katib, A. A. (2020). Clinical research authorships: Ethics and problem-solving. *Canadian Journal of Bioethics (Revue Canadienne de Bioéthique), 3*(3), 118.

Kulig, J. C., & Westlund, R. (2015). Linking research findings and decision makers: Insights and recommendations from a wildfire study. *Society and Natural Resources, 28*(8), 908–917. https://doi.org/10.1080/08941920.2015.1037876

Lee, Y. E. C., Sousa, T. V., Stretton-Smith, P. A., Gold, C., Geretsegger, M., & Baker, F. A. (2022). Demographic and clinical profile of residents living with dementia and depressive symptoms in Australian private residential aged care: Data from the Music Interventions for Dementia and Depression in Elderly care (MIDDEL) cluster randomised controlled trial. *Australasian Journal of Ageing,* 1–10. https://doi.org/10.1111/ajag.13104

Lee, Y.-E. C., Stretton-Smith, P., & Baker, F. A. (2022). The effects of group music interventions in residential aged care for people with dementia and depression from a cluster randomised controlled trial: Perspectives from people with dementia, family members and care home staff. *International Journal of Older People Nursing.* https://doi.org/10.1111/opn.12445

Long, C. R., Stewart, M. K., & McElfish, P. A. (2017). Health research participants are not receiving research results: A collaborative solution is needed. *Trials, 18*(1), 449.

Marin-Gonzalezm, E., Malmusi, D., Camprubi, L., & Borrell, C. (2017). The role of dissemination as a fundamental part of a research project: Lessons learned from SOPHIE. *International Journal of Health Services, 42*(2), 258–276.

McNichol, E., & Grimshaw, P. (2014). An innovative toolkit: Increasing the role and value of patient and public involvement in the dissemination of research findings. *International Practice Development Journal, 4*(1), 1–14. https://doi.org/10.19043/ipdj.41.008

Park, A. L., Kjerstad, E., Crawford, M. J., & Gold, C. (2016). Cost-effectiveness analysis of a randomised controlled trial of improvisation music therapy for young children with autism (TIME-A) in the UK. Post presented at the *Examining the utility of music interventions for children with learning disabilities.* Royal Society of Medicine.

Purvis, R. S., Abraham, T. H., Long, C. R., Kathryn Stewart, M., Warmack, S., & McElfish, P. A. (2017). Qualitative study of participants' perceptions and preferences regarding research dissemination. *AJOB Empirical Bioethics, 8*(2), 69–74. https://doi.org/10.1080/23294515.2017.1310146

Schroter, S., Price, A., Maličky, M., Richards, T., & Clarke, M. (2019). Frequency and format of clinical trial results dissemination to patients: A survey of authors of trials indexed in PubMed. *British Medical Journal Open, 9*(10), e032701. https://doi.org/10.1136/bmjopen-2019-032701

Sethy, S. S. (2020). Responsible conduct of research and ethical publishing practices: A proposal to resolve "Authorship Disputes" over multi-author paper publication. *Journal of Academic Ethics, 18*(3), 283. https://doi.org/10.1007/s10805-020-09375-0

Tamplin, J., & Baker, F. A., Rickard, N., Roddy, C., & MacDonald, R. (2016). A theoretical framework and therapeutic songwriting protocol to promote integration of self-concept in people with acquired neurological injuries. *Nordic Journal of Music Therapy, 25*(2), 111–133. https://doi.org/10.1080/08098131.2015.1011208

Tamplin, J. D., Clark, I. N., Lee, C., & Baker, F. A. (2018). Remini-Sing: A feasibility study of therapeutic group singing to support relationship quality and wellbeing for community-dwelling people living with dementia and their family caregivers. *Frontiers in Medicine: Geriatric Medicine.* https://doi.org/10.3389/fmed.2018.00245

Thompson, Z., Baker, F. A., Clark, I., & Tamplin, J. (2021). Making qualitative interviews in music therapy research more accessible for participants living with dementia—Reflections on development and implementation of interview guidelines. *International Journal of Qualitative Methods, 20.* https://doi.org/10.1177/16094069211047066

World Health Organisation. (2005). *WHO Statement on public disclosure of clinical trial results.* https://www.who.int/news/item/09-04-2015-japan-primary-registries-network

World Medical Association. (2013). World Medical Association Declaration of Helsinki: Ethical principles for medical research involving human subjects. *Journal of the American Medical Association, 310,* 2191–2194.

CHAPTER 11

Innovation, Intellectual Property, and Commercialisation

INNOVATION

The word innovation is derived from the word "innovate" which means to "make changes in something established, especially by introducing new methods, ideas, or products" (Oxford Dictionary, 2011). Innovation is often used within organisational behaviour literature where it suggests a continuous adaptation process to improve efficiencies within an organisation regardless of whether it is a for profit or not-for-profit organisation (Abdul Razak & Murray, 2017). In other words, innovation concerns the development and adoption of new ways of tackling a problem that are *superior* to current approaches. As creative arts therapists, the idea of innovation in a business sense, is somewhat foreign to us. We do not perceive ourselves as innovators, we are therapists that draw on creative arts to promote wellbeing in our clients. And yet, innovation is at the heart of what we do. In essence, we are constantly creating alternative approaches to "mainstream" treatment to solve a clinical or community problem.

I used the term *superior* to other (mainstream) approaches intentionally, and there are several ways new approaches can be superior. First, and perhaps most importantly, the new innovation may be more *effective* than currently existing pharmacological or non-pharmacological approaches. Innovation is always striving to find a better solution to the problem at hand. Together with improved effectiveness, new solutions strive to be more *efficient* and *cost-effective*. In terms of wellbeing outcomes, efficiencies, and costs can be viewed first through the speed of which the health outcome is achieved (does wellbeing occur more quickly with the innovation?), and or second, the intervention arrives at an outcome but is of lower cost than the current approaches to treatment. Even when the innovation may not be quite as effective as an existing approach, if it leads to a more rapid outcome and can be implemented at a lower cost, then it is likely to be viewed more favourably. The increased need for and popularity of embedding health economics outcomes within creative arts therapies trials (Chapter 4) will assist the discipline of creative arts therapies to make a case that is backed with evidence, for the cost-effectiveness of their interventions.

Acceptability of a newly developed creative arts therapy intervention may be a factor in its superiority over existing approaches. Here, the emphasis is more on whether the new approach will be more acceptable to consumers and whether it or its components meet the needs better than the existing approaches. The greater the acceptability, the greater the likelihood of adherence and therefore improved health outcomes. In assessing acceptability, it is important to consider not just the perception of care recipients, but also the perceptions of those creative arts therapists who will deliver the intervention. The multi-faceted construct of acceptability reflects both cognitive and emotional responses to the intervention which can be further divided into prospective (acceptability prior to engaging with an intervention), concurrent (acceptability during participation with an intervention), and retrospective (acceptability after participation) (Sekhon et al., 2017).

When assessing whether a new intervention is superior in acceptability to an existing intervention, Sekhon et al. (2017) proposes that those delivering or receiving the intervention will have:

1. An affective attitude about how they will, are, and were to engage in with the intervention.
2. Perceived burden of participation—that is, the time, cost, and/or cognitive effort involved in engaging with the intervention.
3. Ethicality and Opportunity Cost—this refers to the extent to which the intervention fits well with the individual's value system and what must be sacrificed in terms of benefits and values to engage with the intervention.

4. Intervention Coherence and Effectiveness refer to the extent to which the participant understands how, why, and to what extent the intervention "works".
5. Self-efficacy—concerns the individuals' confidence in their abilities to undertake the tasks required to engage in the intervention.

> *Case Example: Chronic Pain.* In connecting this with the development of new creative arts therapies interventions, let us use an example of chronic pain. Pharmacology dominates this space, with various drugs on the market to manage pain. However, increasingly, people are searching for alternative approaches to manage chronic pain. Their beliefs may be such that they want a more active role in managing their pain other than resorting to a quick, pharmacological "fix". Any non-pharmacological intervention that reduces the level of pain, may lead to reduced dosage of drugs and a potential reduced risk of dependency on drugs to maintain pain-free living. Majore-Dusele and colleagues (2021), developed a dance/movement approach to treat chronic pain. While it is unlikely (although not impossible!), that dance/movement therapy will totally eradicate pain, if it is more acceptable to patients, it is more likely to have high adherence and likely reduce the dose of pain medication use.

Accessibility. Increasing the accessibility of interventions is another aspect of innovation that creative arts therapists may strive to achieve. It is a given that cultural, family context, socioeconomic status, geographical location, sexual orientation, and cognitive/physical/health-related barriers, can limit access to health services, including that of the creative arts therapies. Innovation may occur by initiating small tweaks to existing interventions that enable some sectors of the population access to an intervention that was previously inaccessible. For the creative arts therapies, collectively, we are a relatively small group of therapists compared with other allied health therapies and small compared with the large population of people that may benefit from our services. Further, we are largely located in cities where demand is highest. Innovation occurs when we change our intervention offerings and test their efficacy, accessibility, and scalability so that they can reach more people in need. Considerations may include moving from individual to group therapy, moving from in-person to telehealth modalities, or engaging a train-the-trainer model whereby we use indirect therapy approaches to train non-specialist healthcare providers to use the creative arts therapies in ways to support care (McDermott et al., 2018). COVID-19 is the perfect example of a context that forced clinicians to be innovative and to re-think their models of practice to ensure that those receiving creative arts therapies, were able to continue. Similarly, this occurs in the research context too. A suite of different studies, including HOMESIDE (Baker et al., 2019) responded to this context, testing the impact of and adaption of to creative arts therapies to online delivery (e.g. Garcia-Medrano, 2021; Loi et al., 2022; Re, 2021; Tamplin et al., 2021). In HOMESIDE, we had just begun to implement our "in-person" training program when COVID-19 was first reported. In HOMESIDE, using a train-the-carer model, we provided family carers of people with dementia with training in the use of music therapy informed interventions to support the care of their loved ones with dementia. When COVID-19 pandemic sent the globe into lockdown, we redesigned our intervention to be delivered online via videoconference. Not only did this enable us to continue with our trial, but it also enabled us to reach participants in regional and remote areas that would otherwise never have received such services.

Safety. Improving the safety of interventions is another aspect of innovation that is relevant for the creative arts therapies. We are always advocating that our approaches are safer[1] when compared with pharmacological approaches. Safety links closely with acceptability, as interventions are more likely to be acceptable when shown to be safer than other options.

Intellectual Property—Copyright, Patents, Trademarks, and Secrets

Intellectual property (IP) refers to intangible creations of the human intellect (World Intellectual Property Organisation, 2016). Academics in the creative arts therapies are familiar with the copyright IP attached to their published scholarly works or creative outputs such as artistic works (e.g. paintings), dramatic works, composition, performances, musical recordings or broadcasts, cinematographic and multimedia works, or scientific discoveries. This means that reproduction of this work cannot

---

[1] I use the word safer here as opposed to safe, as inspired by dialogue I had with Art Therapist Jordon Potash who commented that for some people, it will never be safe, but just "safer" than other contexts.

occur by others without fulfilling the specific copyright request processes demanded by the person holding the copyright (which may or may not necessarily be the person who created it). However, there are other forms of IP that may occur as the result of work that creative arts therapy researchers may generate. These include field notes, patentable and non-patentable inventions, registered and unregistered designs, trademarks, databases and software, and any other know-how, trade secrets, and other proprietary information. Let us explore a few of these.

According to the WIPO Intellectual Property Handbook (WIPO, 2013), a patent is a right granted by a government agency to the creator (or their successor-in-title) of an invention or process, which excludes others of the rights to making, using, selling, or importing the invention for a fixed or limited period, in exchange for public disclosure of an invention. The invention is normally a solution to a problem which may be a product or process. Trademarks differ to patents in that they are a recognisable sign, design, or expression which distinguishes it from other products or services. An example is that of a business logo such as our MATCH product (Fig. 11.1). And finally a trade secret is a formula, practice, process, design, pattern, or compilation of information which is not generally known or reasonably ascertainable, by which a business can obtain an economic advantage over competitors and customers (WIPO, 2013). In this sense, the contents of our MATCH carer training package could be considered a "trade secret".

Establishing IP Asset Segments

To track when, where, by whom, and by what means IP has been created, it is important to keep a clear record of any IP created during research. Most universities will have standard IP disclosure forms to complete which will help ensure you are recording the correct information from the get-go. The form serves as a legal record of the IP creation which will be held by the university's legal team on your behalf. As it's a legal document of sorts, it is important to check with all parties involved in the creation of the IP, that they are aware of and agree with the contents of the submission. Typically, the form will contain the following contents:

1. The title of the IP created.

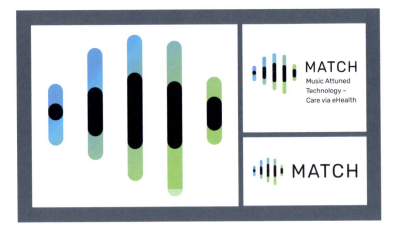

Fig. 11.1 Examples of MATCH trademarked logo

2. The names of people involved in the creation and whether they are (a) the creator, (b) contributor, or (c) student. Creators are defined as any person/s whose input was necessary and would otherwise could not have been created without their input. The creator is defined as anyone who has conceived or contributed to an essential element of the invention, either independently or jointly with others during the evolution of the invention or its reduction to practice. It should be noted that co-authors of publications are not necessarily regarded as creators. Someone listed as a contributor, is a person/s who may have assisted in translating the IP to practice but may not have provided intellectual or creative input of significance.
3. Description of the IP including any documented evidence such as manuscripts, grant applications, validations of its impact from research, and descriptions of prototypes. In addition, the statement should include the "problem" the IP solves, what current solutions (if any) exist, and any advantage your solution offers.
4. Description of the stage of development your IP is currently at. Is it (1) just an idea/concept, (2) in the first stages of development,

(3) proof of concept stage,[2] (4) prototype stage,[3] or (5) minimal viable product.[4]

5. Date when the first IP was created (this could be from notes, experimental data, etc.).
6. For software, detail the use of all open-source code, free executable code, public domain code, and other executable or source code that was not written by the authors.
7. Details of any IP that was in collaboration with other researchers overseas (include date, names of researchers, nature of work performed, and country).
8. Public disclosures—these are details of any aspects of the research that have been publicly disclosed. These could be an online or in print journal, a conference or seminar (abstract and PowerPoint), or conversations. Provide any publication details and the relevance to the IP and state how it differs to the IP created. Make sure to attach any relevant disclosure documents.
9. Provide details of any research grants or contract funds that was used during the development of IP. Details include project start/end dates, co-investigators who are co-applicants, and any sub-contractors.
10. Provide details of future research that will further validate the intellectual property.

---

[2] Proof of concept is a theoretical demonstration of a process/product/concept, which is created to determine whether the idea can be translated into reality. It allows researchers to see whether an idea is viable and to explore its potential. It offers an opportunity to identify any technical or logistical issues that might interfere with its successful development. Proof of concept is not designed to test market demand not what the best production process is. It is the testing of an idea.

[3] Prototype is a very early draft of a process/product/concept that can be tested for usability, functionality, and design. It is not a product that is expected to be "market ready" nor have all the features. Its purpose is to give stakeholders, investors, and users, an idea of what it "might be like" once fully created. Its purpose is to also allow the creators to determine how to best develop the product when it moves into full production.

[4] A Minimal Viable Product (MVP) is a usable version of a product that may contain just the core feature or features, ideal for testing, resulting in feedback and useful data that can be used to shape the first product for sale.

Is Commercialisation a Dirty Word?

In the science, engineering, and technology departments of universities, the concept of commercialisation is a usual part of the day-to-day language and business of academics (Wardle et al., 2019). While they may not have initially set out to commercialise their work, sometimes break through discoveries do occur that can have real-world impact. These breakthroughs can sometimes lead to the commercialisation of outputs, and as such, generate substantial income for the university and for the researcher.

As creative arts therapists, the idea of commercialising our research, is novel and sometimes an uncomfortable thought to hold. After all, there are several tensions between university research and industry research that we must navigate within our psyche so that we become comfortable and open to it (Glenna, 2017). First, university research concerns addressing a societal responsibility in contrast to industry research which is interested in proprietary responsibility. Second, university research focuses on the advancement of knowledge versus the advancement of marketable products and profits which are the concern of industry-based research. Philosophically, university research has open-ended and often long-term goals which contrasts with industry research which explores solutions to short-term, fast, and urgent objectives. In academia, we focus on open communication, sharing our findings, methods, and knowledge widely with the ideal pursuit of extending knowledge being first and foremost in our minds. Again, industry research is more protective, generating knowledge, patents, and processes in secret so that they can have first-to-market advantage over others also working on solutions to the same problem. And finally, university research is disinterested in monetary outcomes whereas industry research expects to generate an income even in those organisations sets up as social enterprise.[5]

These fundamental differences inherently introduce conflict of interest to those wishing to move towards commercialising research (Jukola, 2016). And as such, as researchers we may experience an internal tension. How do we internally rationalise that our work with vulnerable people

---

[5] *Social Enterprises* are an innovative breed of businesses that exist to create a fairer and more sustainable world. They trade to intentionally tackle social problems, improve communities, provide employment, and training or help the environment. The majority use at least 50% of their profits to reinvest in their social mission (Business Victoria, 2021).

may lead to a commercial output further down the track? As a music therapist bound by the Australian Music Therapy Association's code of ethics, it clearly states that we are not to exploit clients. For example, we cannot include testimonials from clients in advertising our music therapy services. Already, I experience tension in this simple yet not so simple scenario. We regularly include participant quotes in the publications of our qualitative studies to show transparency of how researchers arrived at their findings. And yet, we cannot use the same quotes on a webpage to advertise a creative arts therapies service or to advertise participation in a research study. I do not want to go into a dialogue here about the complexities and ethics of this issue, but just to say, that this tradition of not being permitted to use testimonials as evidence of the acceptability of an intervention, has led many researchers to reject the notion that we can commercialise our intellectual property (IP). I too did not enter the world of academia with an intention to commercialise my IP. I was interested in making a long-standing contribution to the evolution of music therapy, and to support the development and refinement of music therapy interventions that would enable vulnerable people to live healthier and happier lives. Once I began creating IP and developing and testing a program that could be potentially scaled up, the university encouraged me to consider taking the creative output down the path of commercialisation. At first, this did not sit comfortably with me, but over time and after talking with many people in the university, I became aware of the fact that for many health researchers at the university, that this was business as usual.

COMMERCIALISING THE CREATIVE ARTS THERAPIES

Like other health disciplines, the commercialisation potential of creative arts therapies research is beginning to gain traction. There is a plethora of opportunities for creative arts therapy researchers to commercialise their research although yet, no discussion of any commercial outcomes has been published. But let us consider a few opportunities yet untapped. First and foremost, we regularly develop and test new creative arts therapy interventions that have the potential to be standardised and widely implemented. When we manualise our interventions for our randomised controlled trials, there is no reason these cannot later be packaged up as a standardised manual that can be published and sold for use by clinicians in the field. These manuals contain detailed guidelines and implementation plans for delivering the intervention as well as methods to assess the effectiveness of them on those clients receiving the intervention (e.g. Baker & Tamplin, 2006; Blomdahl et al., 2022; Carr et al., 2021; Cassity, 1996; Kirkwood et al., 2019).

Another innovation with commercialisation potential that may be created during creative arts therapies research is the development of a diagnostic assessment tool or a novel way of assessing clients. As just one of many examples is the recent development and evaluation of the Movement Assessment and Reporting App (MARA) developed by Dr Kim Dunphy (Schoenenberger-Howie et al., 2022). This technology-based assessment tool was designed for use by dance movement therapists and music therapists to improve accuracy, speed, and feasibility of assessment of clients with intellectual disabilities, children with special needs, in neurological rehabilitation with acquired brain injuries, clients with stroke and spinal cord injuries, dementia, Parkinson's, the mental health sector, family violence, people seeking asylum, and the field of psychiatry and psychosomatics. The International Music Therapy Assessment Consortium was established to support the development of a catalogue of assessment tools in music therapy. Several have been developed. Other examples include the publication of a manual for the Music-Based Scale for Autism Diagnostics (Bergmann et al., 2019), for the Music Therapy Assessment Tool for Awareness in Disorders of Consciousness (MATADOC) 2nd ed. (Magee, 2016), and the Music Attentiveness Screening Assessment—Revised (MARS-R) (Wolfe & Waldon, 2009).

> *Case Study. MATCH.* More recently, together with my research team, we have been developing music-based technological tools to support assessment and intervention for people living with dementia. Our MATCH (Music Attuned Technology—Care via eHealth) project has drawn on our IP developed in HOMESIDE and adapted and extended it to create a commercial output—an integrated eHealth system that embeds music therapy informed principles with sensor technology that is designed for early detection and regulation of agitation in people with dementia. It uses a physiological feedback loop system that interprets, matches, and adapts music to the biobehavioural markers detected in wearable sensors. It also embeds family carer and professional carer training programs that

> teach carers to use music in intentional and mindful ways to support the day-to-day care of people with dementia. Throughout this chapter, I refer to this case study as I outline the many tasks involved in commercialising this research innovation.

Engaging with the Business Development Departments at Universities

As already mentioned, many universities now have well-resourced business development departments that support academics in managing industry engagement, intellectual property, technology transfer, and entrepreneurship initiatives. In various ways, they can assist researchers to leverage intellectual assets and capability and gain a better understanding of how research outcomes can be translated into impactful products beyond the world of academia. The departments can support academics to evaluate the risks and rewards of impact pathways and industry partnerships while also assessing the market readiness of their products. They may provide appropriate legal advice on IP and manage the portfolio of IP assets. Importantly, they may provide continuous and tailored relationship management with new and existing industry partners and with venture capital fund partners. When necessary, they can facilitate the execution of commercial transactions including applying commercial metrics so that the researchers (and university) can receive the best return and impact on their investment. Most of all, the commercialisation department can be wonderfully supportive and encouraging of academics to think beyond the obvious impact.

My experience working within two leading research-focused institutions—The University of Queensland (2002–2012), and The University of Melbourne (2013 to current)—has always been positive when it concerns supporting commercialisation of research. When at The University of Queensland, I was fortunate to engage with Uniquest, a commercial arm of the university. They first opened my eyes to the concept of commercialisation, and at the time I was there, were celebrating the success of commercialising the highly successful and lucrative Triple P program (positive parenting program). Following my move to University of Melbourne, I developed and secured funding for the HOMESIDE carer training program. Once up and running, our university's commercialisation office identified HOMESIDE as having commercial potential. From here, a series of supports were put in place to enable its development and growth. But as business development is not something I have previously had any training in, I was reliant on expertise within the commercialisation office to support me. Developing MATCH from HOMESIDE, was a complex process with several concurrent activities all contributing to its evolution. The first concerns assessing the potential for commercialisation.

ASSESSING COMMERCIAL POTENTIAL OF YOUR IP

Before any researcher (herein founder[6]) embarks on commercialising their IP, they need to assess whether there is a market need and whether there is any value in investing time and energy into commercial development. There are several tasks associated with such assessment but essentially it aims to assess—Who are my customers? What does their job entail? What problem do they have in completing their job that I can solve? What's my product? What features of my product or service address my customers' needs and problems? What is my value proposition?

To answer these questions for assessing the commercial potential of MATCH, my team and I first explored who our "customers" were, we determined what the current problems and personal and financial costs to individual and society were, conducted a market analysis of existing products and then identified local (Australian) and then global markets. We were then able to arrive at our value proposition (Table 11.1).

PRODUCT DEVELOPMENT

After assessing an IP's potential for commercialisation, the next step is to develop it into a product. Dependent upon the type of "product", this could involve a series of steps. For MATCH, one of our first tasks was to break down the very many tasks to product development into different phases. Importantly, we had to separate two not mutually exclusive functions—the technology and business development. To an extent, these two were interdependent, but they were also developed separately and with

---

[6] The Founder is the person/people who create a start-up company and develop the company's vision and business plan.

Table 11.1 Assessment of commercial potential of MATCH

Problem—the need for safe and affordable care of people living with dementia	At the time of writing this chapter, there were 485,000+ Australians living with dementia and 90% of them will present with agitation and other challenging symptoms. This costs the Australian economy nearly AU$15 billion per year to treat. The global cost of the 55 million people living with dementia is estimated at US$818 billion per year. Reducing agitation by small amounts will decrease costs worldwide by 8%. The dementia burden is normally (75% of cases) borne by family carers. Pharmacological treatments are a last course of action for carers and patients because of their harmful side effects. Compounding other problems facing the sector, professional carers experience low job satisfaction, burnout, and high staff turnover and 29% leave the aged care sector
	The onset of agitated behaviours is the result of an escalation in arousal triggered by physical, social, or emotional unmet needs. However, the escalation point is hard for humans to detect until it reaches levels where it leads to negative changes in behaviour. Agitation may continue to worsen until halted by an intervention such as medication. Currently no system exists to detect, monitor, and intervene early to avoid reaching peak levels of agitation

(continued)

Table 11.1 (continued)

Solution	As Music attunement is one of the few evidenced based treatments for agitation, the Australian Royal Commission into aged care recommended aged care providers must offer music therapy by 2024. Our published clinical trial (Baker et al., 2022. The Lancet Healthy Longevity) showed that implementing this recommendation would decrease agitation and reduce care costs by 8%
	And here's why music works: when we listen to familiar music, our bodies and brains synchronise to the beat. For example, music helps maintain cadence when we run. During music attunement, music therapists adapt rhythm and other music components in real time to match a person's biobehavioural markers of agitation, and then gradually adapt the music to regulate them. However, as episodes of agitation can occur at any time, often when clinicians aren't available, an intervention that can replicate this process either by a carer or a technology would go part way to solving this problem
	Our app embeds a series of bespoke training modules that inform carers about how to effectively harness the unique power of music during day-to-day care. Carers are guided to review the training modules that target their own individual needs. For example how to use music to decrease anxiety during showering and dressing tasks
	Biobehavioural markers of agitation are detected through applied wearable sensors and algorithms which then recommend music to MATCH severity of agitation. A closed-loop physiological feedback system adapts music components to match and regulate agitation
Customers	Family carers, residential aged care providers, dementia day centres, geriatric/delirium hospital wards

Competitors	While existing products may seem similar (for confidentiality these competitors have been removed), our product is research backed, safe, embeds carer training, and can detect, monitor, and treat symptoms in real time. Our competitors are merely dementia friendly Spotify like playlists
Value Proposition	MATCH helps families and aged care providers to safely manage symptoms of agitation by offering a clinically tested, effective, low cost integrated system that has been co-designed with our customers
Size of the market	In 2022, there was approximately 8.2 million living with dementia in English speaking countries. The global population is much larger

two different teams. For developing the technology, we separated out the tasks into roles that four separate work teams focused on. Workstream 1—the music therapy content team—were responsible for the design, evaluation, and refinement of the carer training programs (both family and professional carer training), and the recommended music components for the automated system. Here, we used our music therapy informed knowledge, to design a set of rules about which music components should inform which music was best "matched" to different arousal and agitation levels. Workstream 2—human computer interaction team—were responsible for the co-design of the mobile application so that the carer training programs were embedded in an app that had an appealing and understandable interface, and that there was an intuitive logic and flow between sections within the app. Workstream 3 comprised of the software and hardware engineers who were responsible for taking the content developed in workstream 1 and the design features from workstream 2 and program the algorithms that would recommend which music was appropriate for "matching" agitation and adapt it to regulate. Workstream 4 were the clinical team who worked closely with other workstreams to bring the clinical, design, and music therapy content together to ensure that the system could be used in the field.

To make clear the steps needed to develop the technology, a development map was created (Fig. 11.2), which articulated major milestones. However, steps within these were then broken down into smaller tasks, some of which are described below.

Step 1. Translation of IP into a Proof of Concept

The first task is to take the IP you created from your research and translate it into a proof of concept for further research and testing. Dependent upon the degree to which your idea is already developed, you may be at a proof of concept phase aimed at testing the intervention or you may have already completed that stage and are ready to translate it into a potential product (technology, manual, program, etc.). For MATCH, we had already tested the family carer training program in a randomised controlled trial with carers and the people they were caring for (Baker et al., 2019). For us, the first step was to transform this program into a proof of concept for a mobile application. This involved several phases drawing on the skill set of workstreams 1 and 2. Workstream 1 was involved in scripting and filming the training and preparing videos of

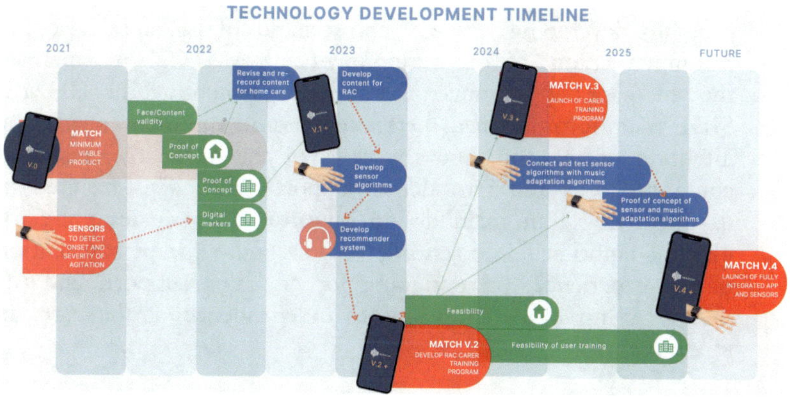

TECHNOLOGY DEVELOPMENT TIMELINE

Fig. 11.2 Technology development timeline

case studies. Meanwhile, workstream 2 worked with a series of phases in developing the prototype:

1. *Identifying key ideas, users, and the market*—we implemented an online survey of both carers of people with dementia and music therapists who had implemented the in-person training program as part of the HOMESIDE randomised controlled trial to gather knowledge about our market and our market needs as well as conducting some online focus groups (during COVID-19 pandemic). For example, we asked questions of the music therapists such as "what value do you expect to add to your users/customers?" "What do you want the ideal product to accomplish?" "How do you imagine your customers would use the product?" "How often would you expect or wish them to use it?". In identifying the market, we explored local (Australian) and global data including the size of the market living at home and those living in residential aged care, the languages spoken, and the geographical location (city, regional, rural). We also undertook the literature reviews to determine the technological capabilities and access to internet that older people report.
2. *Gathering key design requirements*— this involved synthesising existing evidence, observing footage of the in-person carer training

program, developing personas[7] and scenarios of use, and developing recommendations of app requirements. In MATCH, we analysed the video footage of music therapists implementing the HOME-SIDE training program to better understand the users' needs, the intention of the app, and the skills of the music therapist that could be translated into design opportunities. This resulted in us identifying four main design opportunities. (a) designing for physical embodied interactions, (b) designing for personalisation of the experience, (c) designing for empathic support, and (d) designing modules that promotes independence of the carer in music use.

When creating personas representing intended users, we needed to consider both the nature of caregivers, and people with dementia. Carers could be family—partner vs adult child, sibling, friend, the gender of the care partner and the gender of the person with dementia, the age of the person with dementia, and whether they were at early, moderate, advanced stages.

Based on the data available during this phase of gathering key design requirements, it is important that the research team identify and rate the degree of impact for each. This information will inform the next stage in the technology development. For example, one design requirement under embodied interactions was that the research team noted "Body language played a key role in exemplifying how to perform musical activities. In most of the activities, the music therapist modelled body movements that were adopted by the carer and person with dementia. For example, when completing a relaxation exercise, the music therapist relaxed back into the armchair swaying her arms gently to the side. The carer and person with dementia mirrored her relaxed body posture. After the activity, the carer suggested that she enjoyed the activity, and they would not have been able to perform that activity by themselves". This informed the research team

---

[7] A persona is a word used in user-centred design and marketing that describes a fictional character created to represent a user type within the target market. In essence, a persona is a representation of the characteristics and behaviours of the person/s we are designing our product for. In the case of MATCH, different personas were developed for different types of carers of people with dementia—a spouse, an adult child, a sibling, etc. These characteristics help to imagine how, where, why, and in what ways the product will be used by them.

that content needed to have training videos that exemplified how to use embodied interactions for each activity. In terms of the app development, it was important to note that when users are using the app on a smart phone, that the screens may be too small to show clearly how to use body movement and therefore it would be helpful to have the device easily connected to an external display for viewing.

Step 2. Conceptual Design and Development of Low-Fidelity Prototype

After design requirements have been identified, the team began with the development of the conceptual design and *low-fidelity prototype*.[8] Here, the technology is progressed by identifying design solutions and approaches, design patterns and mechanisms of action, concepts to be implemented, task structures, and information architecture. This phase also is used to prepare a scope of work for the technology developers to use in creating a *high-fidelity prototype*.[9] The prototype can comprise of a series of wireframes which are visual representations of a product page. Figure 11.3 illustrates some of the wireframes that formed the initial low-fidelity prototype. Some of these features were later discarded and others added as needed.

Step 3. Iterative Design and Evaluation of High-Fidelity Prototype

The next step in our product development involved an iterative cycle of mobile app design and evaluation. The main aim of this phase was to understand how people living with dementia and their caregivers would value and use the app to support their daily life needs. This was aimed at arriving at a co-designed high-fidelity prototype. In other words, building on the low-fidelity prototype as a starting point that is iteratively developed until we arrive at a high-fidelity prototype. During this stage in the

---

[8] Low-fidelity prototypes are early visual displays of design solutions, which helps the research team to further innovate and improve. As they are usually rough sketches, the team (and those who are reviewing it), usually feel more comfortable making changes to the design at such an early stage. Prototypes do not look and feel like a product, but can provide information on the visual design, the content, and the interactivity (e.g. the flow between screens and sections of the mobile application).

[9] High-fidelity prototypes are computer-based prototypes of the app allowing for realistic user interactions. These take the team as close as possible to a true representation of the user interface.

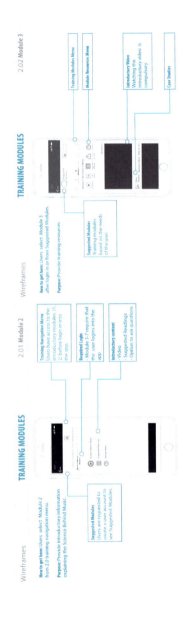

Fig. 11.3 Example of initial wireframes of MATCH

design, we tried to explore any further design requirements that enabled carers to use music in a therapeutically informed way as well as gaining a better understanding of adaptations needed to overcome any technological barriers that we encountered in the co-design workshops with carers.

We utilised a three-cycle participatory action research method starting with workshops with carer participants reviewing the low-fidelity mock-up prototype, and then based on feedback, we began to design and build the *front end*[10] of the app, in collaboration with the technology developers. At this stage, the *back end*[11] had not yet to be developed. Iteratively, we would present various versions of the front-end high-fidelity prototype, to carers who would try it. We would observe their interaction with the prototype and ask for feedback which was used to inform adaptations and refinements.

Step 4. Production and Testing of Minimal Viable Product

Once the prototype has been refined and agreed upon by the team as a minimal viable product (MVP), it can move to the testing phase. A MVP is a fully operating application which contains the most basic or critical set of functions that deems it useful for the user. It is at this point, that the front and back ends of the application need to be connected and operational. When this milestone has been achieved, researchers may use this MVP to perform their initial testing in the field. It is at this point that the research team need to check that their "product or program", achieves what they intended it to do, and that the product is acceptable, accessible, feasible, and useful to the end-users.

In MATCH, once the developers had connected the front and back ends of the mobile app, the research team were ready to test its implementation in a real-world setting. Here, we aimed to:

---

[10] The front end of a technology application consists of everything that the user can view when interacting with a device. This includes components such as a navigation menu, buttons, icons, photographs, embedded videos or podcasts, branding, and text colours and styles.

[11] The back end of a technology application consists to the components of a technology application that operates the application and cannot be accessed by the user. Most data and operating syntax are stored and accessed in the back end of the technology system.

1. Test whether the music intervention training content of MATCH was comprehensible, useful, and adequate for training family carers to use music with people with dementia.
2. Assess the preliminary acceptability, usability, and adherence of use of MATCH by carers.
3. Identify enablers and barriers to adoption and use of MATCH that may inform design modifications.
4. Test the preliminary effectiveness of MATCH use on neuropsychiatric symptoms and agitation of people with dementia.

Using a combination of data collection techniques, we were able to answer these questions and progress towards product refinement to prepare it to be market ready.

Business Development

Alongside the technology development, the team may also begin to prepare a business development plan. Like the technology development, this also involves several steps and tasks which may be being addressed concurrently.

Competitors

As mentioned earlier, an important component of the commercialisation of IP is to review the existing market and explore what the "competitors" are doing. It is important to explore the features of their offerings, their success, the size of the market they currently service, and what their pricing structure is. This analysis helps the research team to identify their value proposition and unique offering. In other words, what makes your product better, or what need does your product serve that existing products do not or do not do adequately.

For MATCH, we evaluated mobile applications that we searched through the Apple Store and Google Play Store using the search terms "dementia, Alzheimer, music and music therapy". Our evaluation showed that most of the apps were providing predominantly music listening and music relaxation activities, and to a lesser extent, singing or support for movement to music. Only a small portion of the applications were designed for people with dementia, the majority were targeting neurotypical older adults. Very few apps contained a music assessment, and/or personalisation of music playlists, and only two provided training within the app. Other features we evaluated included who the developer was (health care, researchers, for profit, not-for-profit), the category the app was assigned to, and what platform (iOS or android) they were available for.

Paths to Commercialisation

Trying to determine what the best path to market is, may be one of the most challenging decisions the research team needs to make. The most popular are (1) creation of a spin-off company, (2) licensing, and (3) sale of the IP/product.

Creation of a spin-off company. Research-based spin-off companies are regarded as the primary approach for launching research informed products to the market. A spin-off company is the creation of an independent company through the sale or distribution of new shares of an existing business or division of a parent company. These spin-offs are expected to be worth more as an independent entity than if it remained as part of a larger business. Building on a spin-off company model is the research spin-off company which belongs to one of the following categories (Callan, 2000):

1. Companies that have an equity investment from a national library or university.
2. Companies that licence technology from a public research institute or university.
3. Companies that consider a university employee to be a founder.
4. Companies that have been established directly by a public research institution.

It is recognised that research-based spin-off companies generate more income for the parent institution than licensing to established companies (Wnuk et al., 2016). However, such spin-offs can be challenging to establish and hold a lot of risk, especially when the product or technology has yet to be proven and not verified by the industry sector. The concept of a spin-off company is exciting to researchers but it does require input from someone with business knowledge, expertise, and a commitment to supporting the initiative from its inception. Wnuk et al. (2016) suggest that success is dependent on the quality of the management.

Licensing. Licensing is another approach to commercialisation which allows individuals or businesses to use a researcher's IP for commercial again in exchange for a fee. To date, this is the most popular approach to commercialisation (Wnuk et al., 2016). The advantage of this approach is that it demands little financial outlay from the licensor (researcher) and therefore carries less risk compared with a spin-off company. The downside to this approach, however, is that the researcher who owns the IP, does lose a degree of control over the use of it.

Sale. Selling the IP is another approach to commercialise and has been said to be the recommended approach when the market has been monopolised and when other forms of commercialisation are not possible (Handler & Burrell, 2005). It generates immediate revenue; however the researcher loses all rights and control over its usage because the IP is transferred on to the buyer (Wnuk et al., 2016). Further, the sale is usually for a fixed price and usually substantially lower than the revenue that would be generated through either a licensing arrangement or spin-off company. The return on investment is "capped" at the agreed price so there are no royalties or bonus payments included if the product becomes hugely successful.

Collaborating with Industry

When beginning the path to commercialisation, the research team need to engage with industry. The industry can be further broken down to different types of stakeholders. First, there are the industry partners who will either purchase, refer or promote the "product" you are commercialising to users (hospitals, advocacy groups, aged care homes, schools), there are the industry partners who may fund the dissemination of the product (private health insurance, government health departments, community centres), and there are the industry partners who may invest or co-produce the product such as technology firms. When considering developing strategic partnerships, Pertuze et al. (2010) recommend the research team consider a number of factors:

1. Identify who are the different types of partners and where they sit within the broad industry context. This can be easier to identify by breaking it down into layers. In Fig. 11.4, I outline the various layers (Fig. 11.4a) and what these layers were for MATCH (Fig. 11.4b).

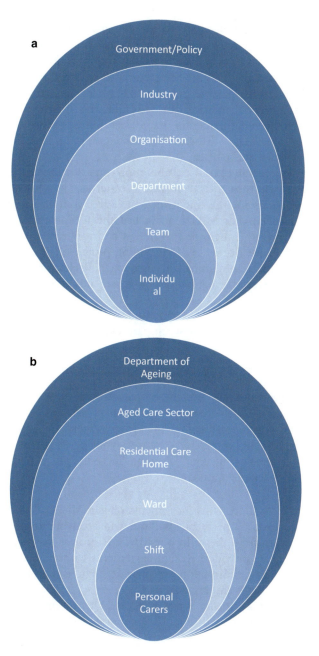

Fig. 11.4 (**a**) Layers of collaborators. (**b**) Layers of collaborators in MATCH

2. Define the context for your partners to ensure there is alignment in vision. It is important at this point to identify what the goals of each partner at each level are, and how can your "product" help them to achieve their goals. Here, the research team need to identify what the problem the partner industry may be facing that your research has the potential to solve. In MATCH, this was to reduce agitation symptoms of dementia, reduce care costs, reduce the number of falls associated with behavioural changes, reduce medication use, and improve quality care.
3. Share your vision of how collaboration can assist the university team but also help their own company. In other words, what do we need as researchers for the initiative to be successful, and what do our partners need? For MATCH, we had the technology-solution but not the investment needed to design and program the software in a way that was market ready including professionally recording the training videos, designing an engaging and elegant interface, and producing wearable hardware that is safe and acceptable to people living with dementia.
4. Invest in establishing good communication to sustain long-term, the emerging relationships between partners and the research team.

Confidentiality Agreements

IP has the potential to be "stolen" by partners and give them a first-to-market advantage. When working with industry partners, it is important to ensure that you prepare confidentiality agreements ahead of revealing any of your IP. This will help to protect your IP from use or misuse by those you are sharing your IP with. There are three types of these agreements dependent upon context.

1. One-way confidentiality agreements refer to the sharing of your IP with an external party but without you receiving any confidential information from them. In our MATCH project, we asked residential aged care providers to sign agreements with us that they would not share any information (or provide demonstrations) about our mobile app with any external party.
2. Mutual Confidentiality Agreements refer to the mutual sharing of your research IP with the IP coming from a potential external

partner. In the case of MATCH, we were interest in a potential collaboration with a technology organisation so we attempted to set-up a two-way confidentiality agreement so that we were protected from the technology company using our IP and vice versa.
3. Multi-Party Confidentiality Agreements are those where the research team may be sharing IP with two or more parties who are also sharing their IP.

Putting the appropriate agreements in place will avoid issues further down the track and ensures you have the appropriate legal requirements in place should a breach of confidentiality occur.

Establishing a New Arm of Your Team

When beginning the commercialisation journey, it is important to recognise what skills you and your team have in this space. In Chapter 4, I discussed assembling a research team. This included creative arts therapy researchers as well as other health and trial related team members (e.g. biostatisticians, trialists, project managers, health economists, etc.). These teams are perfect for implementing a clinical trial. However, when it comes to commercialisation, there is a whole new set of skills that we as creative arts therapy researchers (and the rest of our team), are unlikely to have as it's not been embedded in our training. Some of the skills needed are:

Legal expertise. Legal expertise might be needed for draft and checking amendments made to confidentiality agreements and contracts with industry partners. Appropriate legal advice is needed also for registering the researchers' IP and trademarking any logos or branding. Finally, some products may require approvals from regulatory bodies such as the Food and Drugs Administration (FDA) or country equivalent before it can move to market.

Business development manager. It might be helpful to have an experienced business development manager who is able to help draft the business plan. Their role can be to build a picture of the target market, their relative size, as well as advise the researchers on any relevant aspect of the business. They can help to inform broader decisions such as which market to target first, and when, whether to target the buyer as the individual user, an organisation, or government. They can develop different models of business such as business to business or business to consumer and advise as to which would work best for your product. It is important however, that these business development managers may not know your market as intimately as you do, so the research team should not rely solely on their advice.

A Word of Caution About Commercialisation

When embarking on the commercialisation path, it is important to note that this can become an all-consuming exercise. While my journey towards developing a spin-off company is in its infancy, already I can see ahead of me a choice of whether to completely relinquish my university role and instead, become the chief executive officer of a company of which the university does generate income from. Or do I take a leap of faith, hand the commercialisation of our IP to a separate group of people to run the business. This would mean relinquishing the close control on the product and trusting an experienced business team to take your product and shape it in a direction of their making. At some point, there are just not enough hours in the day to both so as the "inventor", you may need to make a choice. I have not come to that point as I write this chapter, but I can anticipate that it is fast arriving!

Conclusion

While most creative arts therapy researchers are unlikely to commercialise their research, the number that do, is likely to increase with the development of technology and the general increase in acceptance of the value of the creative arts therapies. This chapter, while only touching on some of the issues that affect researchers during the commercialisation process, may provide a frame for those considering following this commercialisation path. While leading a complex team of researchers can be challenging, once legal teams, venture creators, marketers, technology, and business developers are added to the team, the task of bringing people together for a common understanding becomes more challenging. Researchers involved in the development of the IP are more interested in the art and science of the creative arts therapies (as they should be) so have different goals, different timelines to ensure sufficient time and resources are provided to produce the best quality research. This contrasts with the commercialisation team who are more focused on product fit, sale, investors, and accelerating the product's readiness for market. Navigating different ideologies among those two different mindsets and timelines is a never-ending activity.

References

Abdul Razak, A., & Murray, P. A. (2017). Innovation strategies for successful commercialisation in public universities. *International Journal of Innovation Science, 9*(3), 296–314. https://doi.org/10.1108/IJIS-05-2017-0035

Baker, F. A., Bloska, J., Stensæth, K., Wosch, T., Bukowska, A., Braat, S., Sousa, T., Tamplin, J., Clark, I. N., Lee, Y.-E. C., Clarke, P., Lautenschlager, N., & Odell-Miller, H. (2019). HOMESIDE: A home-based family caregiver-delivered music intervention for people living with dementia: Protocol of a randomised controlled trial. *British Medical Journal Open*. https://doi.org/10.1136/bmjopen-2019-031332

Baker, F. A., Lee, Y.-E. C., Sousa, T. V., Stretton-Smith, P. A., Tamplin, J., Sveinsdottir, V., Geretsegger, M., Wake, J. D., Assmus, J., Christian Gold, C. (2022). Clinical effectiveness of Music Interventions for Dementia and Depression in Elderly care (MIDDEL) in the Australian cohort: Pragmatic cluster-randomised controlled trial. *The Lancet Healthy Longevity, 3*(3), e153–e165.

Baker, F., & Tamplin, J. (2006). *Music therapy methods in neurorehabilitation: A clinician's manual*. Jessica Kingsley Publishers.

Bergmann, T., Heinrich, M., Ziegler, M., Dziobek, I., Diefenbacher, A., & Sappok, T. (2019). Developing a diagnostic algorithm for the Music-Based Scale for Autism Diagnostics (MUSAD) assessing adults with intellectual disability. *Journal of Autism and Developmental Disorders, 49*(9), 3732–3752. https://doi.org/10.1007/s10803-019-04069-y

Blomdahl, C., Guregård, S., Rusner, M., & Wijk, H. (2022). Recovery from depression—A 6-month follow-up of a randomized controlled study of manual-based phenomenological art therapy for persons with depression. *Art Therapy: Journal of the American Art Therapy Association, 39*(1), 13–23.

Business Victoria. (2021). *Social Enterprise*. Victorian Government. https://business.vic.gov.au/business-information/start-a-business/business-structures/social-enterprise. Last accessed 8 July 2022.

Callan, B. (2000). Generating spin-offs: Evidence from across the OECD. *STI Review, 26*, 18. https://www.oecd-ilibrary.org/docserver/sti_rev-v2000-1-en.pdf?expires=1658271452&id=id&accname=guest&checksum=1F9F0F15006E1FD29D8457DC49AFAD98. Accessed 20 July 2022.

Carr, C., Feldtkeller, B., French, J., Havsteen-Franklin, D., Huet, V., Karkou, V., Priebe, S., & Sandford, S. (2021). What makes us the same? What makes us different? Development of a shared model and manual of group therapy practice across art therapy, dance movement therapy and music therapy within community mental health care. *The Arts in Psychotherapy, 72.*

Cassity, M. (1996). *Multimodal psychiatric music therapy for adults, adolescents, and children: A clinical manual.* MMB Music.

Garcia-Medrano, S. (2021). Screen–bridges: Dance movement therapy in online contexts. *Body, Movement & Dance in Psychotherapy, 16*(1), 64–72.

Glenna, L. L. (2017). AFHVS 2017 presidential address: The purpose-driven university: The role of university research in the era of science commercialization. *Agriculture and Human Values, 34*(4), 1031–1021. https://doi.org/10.1007/s10460-017-9824-6

Handler, M., & Burrell, R. (2005). *Commercialisation and management of intellectual property: Guidelines for researchers and research managers: A report for the Rural Industries Research and Development Corporation.* Rural Industries Research and Development Corporation. https://www.agrifutures.com.au/wp-content/uploads/publications/05-005.pdf. Accessed 20 July 2022.

Jukola, S. (2016). The commercialization of research and the quest for the objectivity of science. *Foundations of Science, 21*(1), 89–103.

Kirkwood, J., Graham-Wisener, L., McConnell, T., Porter, S., Reid, J., Craig, N., Dunlop, C., Gordon, C., & Thomas, D., Godsal, J., & Vorster, A. (2019). The MusiQual treatment manual for music therapy in a palliative care inpatient setting. *British Journal of Music Therapy, 33*(1), 5–15.

Loi, S. M., Flynn, L., Cadwallader, C., Stretton-Smith, P., Bryant, C., & Baker, F. A. (2022). Music and psychology and social connections program: Protocol for a novel intervention for dyads affected by younger-onset dementia. *Brain Sciences, 12*(4), 503. https://doi.org/10.3390/brainsci12040503

Magee, W. L. (2016). *Music Therapy Assessment Tool for Awareness in Disorders of Consciousness (MATADOC)* (2nd ed.). Royal Hospital for Neuro-disability.

Majore-Dusele, I., Karkou, V., & Millere, I. (2021). The development of mindful-based dance movement therapy intervention for chronic pain: A pilot study with chronic headache patients. *Frontiers in Psychology, 12*(12), 587923. https://doi.org/10.3389/fpsyg.2021.587923

McDermott, O., Ridder, H. M. O., Stige, B., Ray, K., Wosch, T., & Baker, F. A. (2018). Indirect music therapy practice and skill-sharing for dementia care. *Journal of Music Therapy.* https://doi.org/10.1093/jmt/thy012

Oxford dictionary of English (electronic resource). (2011).

Pertuze, J. A., Calder, E. S., Greitzer, E. M., & Lucas, W. A. (2010, January 1). Best practices for industry-university collaboration: Universities can be major resources in a company's innovation strategy. *MIT Sloan Management Review, 51*(4), 83–95.

Re, M. (2021). Isolated systems towards a dancing constellation: Coping with the Covid-19 lockdown through a pilot dance movement therapy tele-intervention. *Body, Movement and Dance in Psychotherapy, 16*(1), 9–18.

Schoenenberger-Howie, S. A., Dunphy, K. F., Lebre, P., Schnettger, C., Hillecke, T., & Koch, S. C. (2022). Die Movement Assessment and Reporting App (MARA) in der Musiktherapie. *GMS Journal of Arts Therapies, 4*. https://doi.org/10.3205/jat000018

Sekhon, M., Cartwright, M., & Francis, J. J. (2017). Acceptability of healthcare interventions: An overview of reviews and development of a theoretical framework. *BMC Health Services Research, 17*, 88. https://doi.org/10.1186/s12913-017-2031-8

Tamplin, J. T., Morris, M. E., Baker, F. A., Sousa, T., Haines, S., Dunn, S., Tull, V., & Vogel, A. P. (2021). ParkinSong Online: Protocol for a telehealth feasibility study of therapeutic group singing for people with Parkinson's disease. *British Medical Journal Open, 11*, e058953. https://doi.org/10.1136/bmjopen-2021-058953

Wardle, J. L., Baum, F. E., & Fisher, M. (2019). The research commercialisation agenda: A concerning development for public health research. *Australian and New Zealand Journal of Public Health, 43*(5), 407–409. https://doi.org/10.1111/1753-6405.12930

WIPO. (2013). *Intellectual property handbook: Policy, law and use.* Chapter 2: Fields of Intellectual Property Protection. https://web.archive.org/web/20130520221306/http://www.wipo.int/export/sites/www/about-ip/en/iprm/pdf/ch2.pdf. Accessed 8 July 2022.

Wnuk, U., Mazurkiewicz, A., & Poteralska, B. (2016). Commercialisation strategies: Choosing the right route to commercialise your research results. *Proceedings of the European Conference on Innovation & Entrepreneurship*, 869–875.

Wolfe, D. E., & Waldon, E. G. (2009). *Music attentiveness screening assessment-revised*. American Music Therapy Association.

World Intellectual Property Organization (WIPO). (2016). *Understanding Industrial Property*. World Intellectual Property Organization. https://doi.org/10.34667/tind.36288. ISBN 9789280525939. Accessed 8 July 2022.

Index

A

Adherence, 8, 33, 37, 50, 60, 85, 87, 117, 160, 163, 172, 183, 186–188, 197, 198, 200, 202, 204, 213, 215, 216, 248, 268

Adverse events
  collection, 69, 87, 157, 177
  forms, 145
  monitoring, 53, 61, 153, 157, 174
  reporting, 53, 158

Art therapy, 12, 42, 164, 174, 186, 189, 202, 203, 230

Assessment, 10, 19, 21, 26–28, 32–36, 39, 42, 49, 50, 54, 62, 66, 67, 70, 87, 98, 100, 113, 130, 152, 159, 160, 169, 170, 172, 173, 176, 177, 185, 188, 198, 200, 201, 203, 212, 214, 226, 242, 256, 258, 268

Assessor, 10, 19, 26, 27, 33, 34, 39, 62, 66, 95, 98, 115, 152, 154, 157, 159, 169, 170, 178, 238

Attrition, 37, 144, 145

Authorship, 14, 60, 89, 224, 235–241, 243

B

Bias, 57, 77, 83, 92, 161, 186, 200, 209, 216, 218, 225, 242, 243

Biomarkers, 87, 157, 159

Biostatisticians, 6, 9, 10, 21, 23, 42, 57, 61–63, 83, 92, 93, 100, 109, 110, 210, 273

Blinding, 157

Budget, 7, 13, 20, 27, 28, 40, 42–44, 50, 53, 55, 56, 58, 59, 84, 87–89, 91, 93, 95, 107–109, 111–114, 116–119, 137, 141, 153, 154, 162, 194, 199

Burden, 12, 14, 72, 73, 125, 128–131, 138, 140–142, 248, 259

Business development, 21, 23, 257, 258, 268, 274

C

Capacity building, 5, 21, 24, 64, 67, 68, 233
Case Report Forms (CRF), 21, 32, 33, 157, 159, 161, 169, 175, 176
  electronic case report forms, 159
Chief investigator, 6, 17, 39, 41, 42, 48, 51, 52, 54–58, 60, 62, 64, 67, 68, 88, 90, 112, 170, 174, 237, 240, 241
Clinical Trials Unit, 48, 50
Collaboration, 8, 12, 68, 72, 76, 89, 90, 143, 199, 253, 267, 272, 273
Collaborators, 89, 235
Commercialisation, 14, 20, 21, 173, 254–258, 268, 270, 273, 274
Commitment, 22, 23, 28, 42, 48, 55, 58, 64, 76, 77, 89, 96, 117, 122, 130, 131, 140, 144, 145, 188, 191, 269
Co-morbidity(ies), 125, 126
Confidentiality, 74, 127, 157, 272, 273
Consent, 10, 38, 124, 128, 130, 137, 143, 154, 155, 169, 228, 235
CONSORT, 172
Conversion, 137, 140
COVID-19, 9, 19, 39, 62, 99, 144, 176, 235, 250, 263

D

Dance/movement therapy, 12, 39, 115, 174, 184, 186, 249
Data
  analysis, 26, 90, 93, 166, 237
  cleaning, 14, 157, 164, 165, 210
  collecting, 10, 14, 25, 33, 34, 36, 38, 70, 90, 93, 94, 99, 107, 110, 113, 131, 144, 151, 153, 154, 156, 157, 160, 161, 175–178, 217, 236, 268
  missing, 14, 28, 38, 62, 63, 69, 94, 95, 116, 117, 152, 153, 158, 159, 161, 164, 176, 210, 214–219
  monitoring, 20, 25, 54, 60, 93, 117, 151, 153, 172
  repository, 173
  security, 14, 157, 163, 169
  sharing, 111, 158, 169, 173
  storage, 53, 156, 157, 159, 163, 170, 173
Database, 6, 14, 22, 26, 27, 32, 38, 69, 89, 94, 95, 102, 111, 113, 116, 117, 132, 134, 135, 153, 155, 157–159, 162–164, 170, 175, 176, 178, 179, 236, 251
  access, 38, 117, 170
  backup, 159
Database management systems, 158
Data base manager, 176
Data entry
  development, 113
  standardisation, 200
  training, 113
Data Management Plan (DMP), 14, 151, 154, 156, 157, 159, 161–163, 169, 170, 173, 174, 214
Data safety and monitoring, 29
Data Safety Monitoring Board (DSMB), 19, 54, 59–63, 67, 69, 93, 110, 116, 153, 178, 211
Declaration of Helsinki, 151, 223
Demographics, 25, 62, 63, 219, 228
Dissemination, 14, 20, 32, 54, 56, 65, 70, 74, 88, 118, 223–226, 228–231, 235, 242, 270
Drama therapy, 12, 186
Dropouts, 60

E

eHealth, 11, 86–88, 141, 160, 173, 174, 256
Electronic data capture (EDC), 33, 115, 158, 159, 161, 162, 165, 169, 175
Eligibility, 32, 114, 123, 144, 213
Eligible, 35–37, 39, 55, 112, 114, 122, 123, 130, 137, 140, 172, 236
Endpoint, 92, 213
Engagement, 29, 68, 70, 71, 75, 115, 118, 127, 130, 131, 133, 145, 160, 187, 201–203, 213, 257
Enrolment, 22, 30, 35, 36, 38, 40, 93, 100, 109, 113, 135, 137, 139, 140, 142, 143, 155, 158, 172, 176, 240
Ethical, 29, 30, 47, 49, 53, 54, 60, 71, 91, 107, 115, 121, 151, 156, 196, 223, 235
Ethical considerations, 31
Ethics, 7, 13, 21, 23, 26, 29, 35, 40, 52, 53, 55, 56, 61, 63, 64, 74, 78, 90–92, 111, 113, 126, 154, 155, 255
Ethics review panels, 48, 74, 211
External validity, 127, 183

F

Feasibility, 4, 8, 10, 11, 21, 30, 36, 49, 70, 85, 87, 108, 160, 256
Feasible, 9, 36, 43, 44, 50, 85, 87, 107, 158, 161, 162, 236, 267
Fidelity, 3, 9, 14, 28, 29, 33, 37, 50, 65–67, 86, 96, 113, 127, 154, 160, 169, 177, 183–187, 189, 190, 193, 194, 197–200, 204, 226, 238, 239, 265, 267
Funding, 1, 3, 4, 9, 20, 36, 41–43, 50–53, 56, 68, 70, 73, 78, 83, 84, 89, 91, 107, 109, 110, 114, 118, 121, 186, 199, 229, 231, 242, 257
Funds, 6, 43, 49–51, 89, 107, 116, 119, 137, 253, 270

G

Gantt chart, 21
General Data Protection Regulation (GDPR), 163, 164
Good clinical practice, 47, 56, 91, 151, 156

H

Harm, 34, 35, 37, 39, 196
Harmful, 122, 138, 193, 259
Health conditions, 75, 125, 126, 145
Health economics, 50, 93, 227, 239, 248
Health economist, 6, 9, 10, 21, 69, 86, 88, 93, 170, 273
Health status, 77, 125, 126, 130, 144, 145
HOMESIDE, 2, 6, 10, 11, 19, 24–27, 39, 40, 42, 43, 52, 55, 62–66, 70–72, 74, 77, 78, 84, 98–102, 109, 111–114, 117, 118, 128, 130, 132–137, 144, 154, 165, 170, 171, 176–179, 188, 190, 195, 198, 201, 204, 212–214, 216, 217, 219, 250, 256–258, 263, 264

I

Imputation, 218
Inclusion, 23, 31, 38, 91, 111, 123, 125, 172, 243
Industry partners, 29, 39, 49, 69, 74, 89, 109, 229, 239, 257, 270, 272, 273
Informed consent, 31, 73, 113, 114, 128, 143, 154, 228

Innovation, 14, 122, 247–250, 256, 257
Intellectual property (IP), 14, 20, 21, 49, 51, 52, 67, 89, 173, 250, 253, 255, 257
Intention to treat, 69, 172, 219
Interdisciplinary, 1, 3, 5, 6, 8, 11–13, 21, 57, 83, 186, 230, 236
Interim reports, 90
Internal validity, 183, 185
Interventionists, 29, 66, 67, 93, 99, 170, 178, 187, 190–192, 195–197, 199, 200, 238
Intervention(s), 2, 3, 5, 8–10, 12, 19, 25–29, 33, 34, 37, 39, 52, 53, 56, 64, 65, 67, 68, 75, 77, 79, 84, 85, 87, 90, 92, 93, 95, 96, 99–101, 108, 109, 113, 117, 122, 124, 126, 127, 130, 139, 142, 144, 154, 156, 157, 160, 167, 169–172, 174, 177, 178, 183–191, 193–204, 212, 214, 216, 226–229, 233, 238, 248–250, 255, 256, 259, 262
Interviews, 2, 74, 117, 132, 135, 157, 226
Investigators
 categories, 101, 174
 manuals, 32, 52
 meetings, 22, 23, 25, 56–58, 61, 64, 76, 90, 102, 118
 recruitment, 20, 38, 59, 60, 64, 113
 relations, 23, 102, 211
 responsibilities, 28, 30, 36, 41, 48, 53, 61, 90, 97, 113, 224
 retention, 90
INVOLVE, 72, 76

K
Kick-off meetings, 64

Knowledge translation, 14, 118, 224, 229, 243

M
Manual of operational procedures (MOP), 29, 32, 91, 156
Manuals, 13, 152, 162, 194, 203, 238, 255, 256, 262
MAPS, 12, 28, 73, 85, 199, 262
Masking, 154
MATCH, 5, 11, 20, 21, 24, 32, 38, 40–42, 44, 51–53, 55, 58, 64, 65, 67, 70, 86, 97, 110, 115, 141, 145, 160, 173, 175, 211, 214, 231, 240, 251, 252, 258–262, 264, 266–268, 270–273
Mechanisms, 2, 35, 55, 56, 59, 68, 156, 159, 160, 174, 203, 223, 265
Medical Research Council, 9, 17, 50, 54, 56
MIDDEL, 10, 19, 29, 33, 35, 36, 38, 64, 109, 110, 114, 115, 137–139, 152, 154, 185, 195, 198, 203, 211, 218, 226, 228, 232, 234
Monitoring, 13, 14, 20, 22, 25, 31, 32, 38, 41, 44, 49, 53, 54, 60, 61, 67, 68, 78, 86, 91, 93, 95, 108, 116, 117, 124, 135, 137, 146, 151–159, 161, 172, 174, 175, 184, 194, 196, 197, 199, 200, 202, 203
 enrolment, 22, 135, 172
 quality, 13, 91, 112, 116
Motivation, 124, 125, 139, 146, 225
Music therapy, 1, 5, 8–12, 21, 39, 51, 67, 68, 73, 83, 85, 86, 95, 97, 115, 143, 190, 203, 226, 233, 234, 250, 255, 256, 260, 262, 268

N

National Institute for Health Research (NIHR), 50, 72, 135

O

Open access, 118, 119, 174, 223, 241, 243
Outcome measures, 10, 33, 62, 69, 84, 115, 161, 165, 169, 170, 172, 177, 188, 210, 217, 236
Outcomes, 1, 3, 6, 10, 13, 25, 49, 54, 56, 59, 61, 72, 75, 76, 84, 86, 93, 96, 107, 110, 121, 124, 126, 139, 160, 161, 174, 183, 185, 188, 189, 193, 197, 200, 204, 209–211, 213, 217, 224–228, 233, 248, 254, 255, 257

P

Participants
  confidentiality, 53, 126, 157
  follow-up, 14, 117, 172
  manual, 211
  modes of contact, 235
  non-compliance, 37
  payment, 142, 145
  recruitment, 14, 38, 61, 65, 91, 95, 111, 114, 115, 121, 131, 153, 213
  retention, 14, 121, 123, 172
  screening, 114, 123, 139, 157, 213
  treatment adherence, 160
  withdrawals, 62, 144, 172, 213
Partner, 12, 21, 40, 111, 128, 138–140, 199, 229, 264, 270, 272
Partnership, 39, 40, 79, 139, 257, 270
Per-protocol, 37, 69, 172, 199
Pilot, 4, 8, 36, 38, 75, 108, 113, 122, 123
Planning phase, 20, 36, 55, 93, 119, 163
Principal investigator, 5, 13, 14, 17–23, 25, 28, 29, 32, 36, 38, 39, 42, 53–59, 61–64, 67, 68, 76, 86, 88–91, 95, 97, 101–103, 110, 111, 119, 163, 174, 177, 212, 217, 239
Product, 21, 41, 131–133, 174, 224, 225, 231, 251, 253, 254, 257, 258, 261–265, 267–270, 272, 274
Project grant/funding, 41
Project management, 6, 13, 14, 18, 20, 28, 29, 43, 44, 112, 118
Project manager, 17, 18, 21–24, 27–29, 32, 36, 41, 48, 51, 54, 67, 69, 86, 89–92, 95, 97, 109, 112, 116, 118, 273
Promotional material, 14, 132, 134, 137, 139
Protocol
  adherence, 22, 91, 154
  contents, 21, 188, 194
  deviations, 61, 116, 197, 213, 215
  violations, 37, 38, 60, 154, 212
Public and patient involvement (PPI), 13, 70, 118, 229
Publication(s), 1–3, 14, 21, 26, 30, 31, 52, 54, 57, 60, 64, 78, 91, 112, 118, 160, 216, 223, 224, 226, 227, 232, 235, 238–243, 252, 253, 255, 256

Q

Qualitative data, 2, 7, 65, 74, 117, 177
Quality of life, 9, 10, 124
Quantitative data, 8

R

Randomisation, 3, 28, 91, 92, 95, 98, 110, 117, 129, 136, 138, 157, 169, 171, 177, 212, 215
  blocked, 92
Randomised controlled trials, 6, 8–10, 12, 52, 64, 67, 84, 108, 122, 123, 130, 133, 169, 172, 185, 198, 215, 255, 262, 263
Recruitment strategy, 7, 14, 25, 28, 37, 38, 42, 43, 71, 122, 124, 131, 132, 136, 137, 146
REDCap, 21, 27, 117, 158, 170, 171, 176, 177, 179
Regulatory approval processes, 107
Regulatory processes, 13, 40, 112, 113
Reporting, 14, 20, 22, 37, 49, 53, 61, 68, 88, 93–96, 102, 116, 151, 154, 156, 158, 172–174, 185–187, 202, 210, 228, 237
Reports, 8, 20, 22, 24, 48, 54, 58, 60–63, 78, 91, 95, 102, 107, 112, 113, 116, 118, 121, 129, 158, 171, 174, 178, 186, 200, 217, 223, 228, 233, 237, 243
Research waste, 6, 20, 107, 121
Resources, 5, 6, 9, 13, 18, 22, 23, 27, 32, 34, 38, 40, 42–44, 55, 76, 77, 83, 85, 93, 107–109, 111, 114, 122, 127, 136, 137, 140, 154, 187, 199, 204, 211, 228, 236, 274
Risk management, 13, 37, 39, 40, 49, 51

S

Safety, 20, 31, 34, 39, 47, 54, 59–62, 70, 87, 98, 124, 127, 138, 153, 158, 214, 250
Sample size, 1, 9, 35, 36, 42, 69, 92, 102, 109, 121–123, 158, 185, 211, 212, 217, 218
Screening, 27, 34, 100, 114, 138, 158, 169, 171, 176
Sponsor, 31, 37, 47, 48, 52, 61, 223
Statistical analysis plan (SAP), 14, 29, 54, 69, 88, 92, 93, 110, 117, 209–216, 219
Strategy, 7, 23, 37, 48, 49, 56, 60, 63, 68, 87, 90, 99, 102, 122, 123, 132, 134–136, 138–141, 145, 146, 154, 176, 184, 194, 202, 204, 224, 228, 231, 232, 239
Study protocol, 13, 19, 29, 30, 32, 33, 60, 69, 92, 93, 111, 136, 156, 160, 209, 212, 226, 236
Study Within A Trial (SWAT), 54, 122, 136

T

Trial, 2–4, 6, 7, 9, 10, 13, 14, 17, 18, 20, 22, 25, 27–34, 36–38, 40, 41, 43, 44, 47–52, 54–61, 63, 65–69, 71, 73, 77–79, 83, 86, 90–94, 98–100, 107–109, 111, 113–118, 121–125, 127, 129, 130, 134, 136–138, 140–144, 146, 151–154, 156, 158, 159, 161, 162, 164, 170, 174, 178, 183, 184, 186, 194, 196, 197, 199, 201, 203, 204, 209, 211–213, 215, 216, 223–225, 227, 228, 231, 248, 250, 260
Trial Management Group (TMG), 48, 54–56, 59, 61, 64, 66, 67, 153, 178
Trial Steering Committee (TSC), 54–61, 118, 153, 178
Trust, 97, 98, 127, 140, 143

Trustworthy/trustworthiness, 108, 152, 160, 164, 209, 215

W
Withdraw, 37, 144
Withdrawal, 31, 62, 157, 213
World Health Organisation (WHO), 35, 223

Printed in the United States
by Baker & Taylor Publisher Services